Human Services

The Third Revolution In Mental Health

Human Services

Alfred Publishing Co., Inc., New York

Alfred
PUBLISHERS

The Third Revolution In Mental Health

Walter Fisher

Joseph Mehr

Philip Truckenbrod

Library of Congress Catalog Card Number: 74-75481

ISBN: 0-88284-013-4

Printed in the United States of America

Alfred Publishing Co., Inc.
75 Channel Drive
Port Washington, New York 11050

PRODUCTION CREDITS

Book Design and Production: Sidney Solomon

Cover Art: Peter Landa

Picture Research: Peter Landa and Raymond Solomon

Composition and Mechanicals: Hubert Carter

Printing: Noble Offset Printers

Binding: Book Press

To The Human Service Warriors

The following is not intended to be a complete list of persons who have contributed to the development and implementation of the human service model. Rather, these are the persons we have drawn from in our conceptual growth and as points of reference in the preparation of this text. We have purposely chosen the label "human service warrior" because it is felt that the struggle to establish pragmatic, problem-solving approaches to the needs of persons in trouble involves struggle and conflict.

Robert Agranoff
George Albee
Saul Alinsky
David Bazalon
Peter Breggin
Franklin Chu
Natalie Davis
Herman Deisenhaus
George DeJong
George Drain
Arthur Dykstra
George Fairweather
Don Fisher
Zoltan Fuzessery
Alan Gartner
J. Douglas Grant
Norris Hansell

Del Hicks
Nicholas Hobbs
Donald Huller
Ivan Illich
Vernon James
Geri Joseph
Myrna Kassel
John F. Kennedy
Ken Kesey
Martin Luther King, Jr.
Ronald Leifer
Neil Mahoney
Mildred McKinny
Harold McPheeters
Walter F. Mondale
Loren Mosher

O.H. Mowrer
Ralph Nader
Arthur Pearl
Charles Percy
Steve Pratt
Julian Rappaport
Frank Reissman
Barbara Seaman
Barry Sugarman
Thomas Szasz
E. Fuller Torry
Sharland Trotter
John True
Harold Visotsky
Roger Wyatt
Philip Zimbardo

And the human service workers who are involved in pragmatic problem-solving in the field.

Contents

Part I
Problems and Issues
in the Human Services Field

Part II
The Traditional
Mental Health Model

Part III
Critical Mass

Part IV
The Human Service Model

Part V
A Glance
Into the Future

Preface

We would first like to express our gratitude to Irene Fisher, Nancy Mehr, and Joan Truckenbrod for their tolerance, ideas, and support for this book, which enabled us to complete its preparation in a little over six months. We would also like to thank Dorothy Lund and Imojean Deibert, both of whom spent many long hours of their personal time transforming our original handwritten copy into a finished manuscript. In addition, we would like to express our intellectual debt to Robert Agranoff and many others of those named as human service warriors on our dedication page. Lastly, to our editor, Roy Grisham, our gratitude for innumerable contributions in organizing and focusing our ideas into its present form.

Walter Fisher
Joseph Mehr
Philip Truckenbrod

October, 1973
Elgin State Hospital
Elgin, Illinois

Human Services

The Third Revolution In Mental Health

Introduction

*I*t is, of course, difficult, if not impossible, to describe the attitudes, values, emotional condition, expectancies, and beliefs of a nation, either briefly or in terms of a number of volumes. In this sense, if one attempted to describe or define the American condition in a paragraph, it would be more of an effort to provide the current flavor rather than the true configuration of the nation.

At this point in history there appear to be certain adjectives, concepts, and themes that continuously appear in the news media and perhaps reflect the current flavor of America: Watergate, corruption, television, immediate information, deviance, informational shock, energy crisis, civil rights, inflation, recession, insecurity, violence, massive insight, cynicism, and lack of trust. A semantic analysis of these terms would quickly and clearly demonstrate that at present, the American life space—the environment in which we live—has more negative than positive overtones.

It is difficult to say whether Western society is literally "going to hell" and disintegrating before its citizens' eyes or whether the massive informational input of newspapers, radio, and, of course, television has created informational shock. In either event, most of us are massively aware that our traditional social institutions are malfunctioning. Not only are most people becoming distrustful and cynical about the traditional social institutions such as marriage, family, and church, but they are now aware that the support and backup social institutions such as mental hospitals, law enforcement, penology, special education, and public aid, are unable to deliver effective social services.

It has long been held by psychoanalysts and therapists in general that insight is the source, or genesis, of growth. If this is true, then the United States is on the threshold of a great new era. The Watergate events, the investigations and the public hearings, have climaxed this informational revolution in the United States, and social scientists will have the opportunity to study the impact of this massive informational input.

In the midst of this turmoil, distrust, insight, and cynicism there appears to be a new enterprise developing in the United States which has been aptly named "human services." This human service movement appears to be budding in almost all of the 50 states and in most of the service fields—mental health, penology, public aid, law enforcement, religion, education, and public affairs. It is not easy to define the concepts or boundaries of the human services enterprise; in fact, it would take this entire book to characterize the new movement. It can be said, however, that this approach has emerged as one antidote to the stress and turmoil in the American society. It is the primary purpose of this book to attempt to bring together many of the human service events budding around the country and provide a crystallization of this movement.

The authors struggled for many weeks with the task of how to present this model. There are a number of issues and problems:

1. It is a recent movement, and there is little research or evaluative material.

2. It has a "pop culture" quality, in that it is constantly changing and growing.

3. It touches so many different disciplines and yet appears to be qualitatively different from any of the individual disciplines or the

summation of the various fields. It represents a new configuration (a new gestalt).

4. The difference between this orientation and other service systems appears to be more attitudinal, or in levels of awareness or consciousness. This is more difficult to define and describe than informational or skill differences.

With these problems in mind, it initially seemed appropriate to present the overall philosophies, ideologies, and beliefs of the human service model, then discuss it in the context of the many relevant service fields. This quickly proved to be an enormous undertaking. The attempt to redefine and reexamine all the human service areas in this new context would take a number of volumes and perhaps several occupational lifetimes.

After this struggle over the content of the book, the task was redefined. It still appeared appropriate to discuss the overall philosophies, ideologies, beliefs, and methods of the human service model, but it was now clearly impossible to describe in detail in one volume all of the disciplines involved in the human service movement. Thus, in addition to discussing the human service movement, the authors decided to discuss human services as a factor in social change and to examine one service system—mental health—in depth. The concepts, themes, and ideologies emerging from this examination are congruent and relevant to the other disciplines, professions, and fields of expertise. The mental health field was selected for two reasons: it is the primary expertise of the authors, and currently most students in the human service field are majoring in mental health.

The book is organized in five parts. In Part I the major problems and issues in the human service field are identified and defined. In Part II the traditional mental health service—the medical model—is described and defined. In Part III the limitations and failures of the traditional system are described in the context of a changing society. Part IV presents the human service model theoretically and concretely as an alternative to the traditional approach. In Part V the human service model is presented as the genesis of a new profession, a new model, and a new level of consciousness.

Part I

Problems and Issues in the Human Services Field

Chapter 1 *Goals and Objectives*

Our purpose in this book is to describe and define an emerging field of knowledge and activity—the *human services*. The importance, impact and immense growth of this field are evident in the development of over 200 human service college programs in less than a decade.

In the field of mental health there has been a radical change since the end of World War II. Although the groundwork for change was laid in the late 1940s and early 50s, significant change came in the late fifties and early sixties. Nicholas Hobbs (1964) has called this radical change—with its new theories, service delivery, and treatment—mental health's *third revolution*.

The revolution in mental health is an important factor in the development of the human services. In addition, a new profession

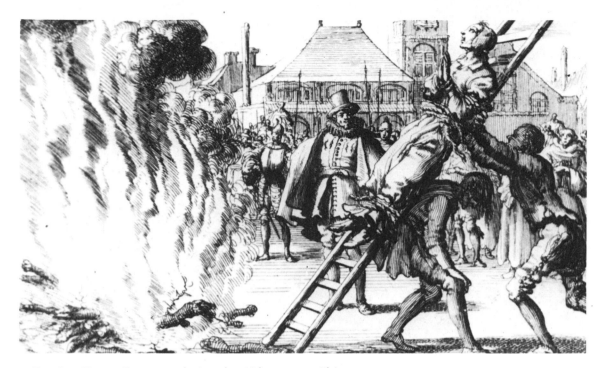

Burning "insane" women during the 16th century. This copper engraving is no exaggeration of the kind of treatment administered for atypical and maladaptive behavior. (Courtesy The Bettmann Archive.)

The *Convulsionaries* (*convulsionaries* of St. Medard, a cemetery of Paris.) The Great Treatment (*grand secour*). The patient stricken by convulsions is subjected to the most atrocious treatment—he is beaten with heavy wooden sticks and tramped on by a number of persons. Copper engraving by B. Picart, *Cérémonies et Coutumes de tous les Peuples.* (Courtesy The Bettmann Archive.)

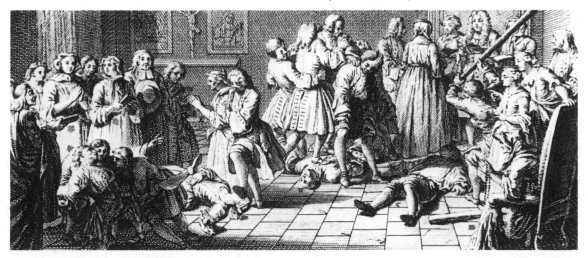

has come into being, which we will call the *human service worker,* or the *generalist.*

The First Revolution or Wave

In order to provide a setting for our discussion, we must give a brief history of the study and treatment of mental disorders. There have been three major revolutions or waves in the field of mental health. The first, which occurred at about the end of the 18th century, has been designated by Gregory Zilboorg (1941) as the beginning of modern psychiatry. Prior to this time, deviant behavior was thought to be a function of witchcraft or sin. If one started with these assumptions, then the burning and killing of deviant people does not seem farfetched. In fact, for a good portion of man's history, the unusual, atypical, eccentric and maladaptive people, particularly the poor and uninfluential, were severely punished, if not executed, for their deviant behavior.

The mental health revolution of the late 18th century reflected the times—the American and French Revolutions, the Declaration of Independence, and the writings of the French philosophers—in all of which it was believed that man was noble and capable of unlimited growth, love and self-actualization. People were different because their education was different. The newborn child, if not encumbered by the evils of civilization, was still capable of realizing his full potential as a human being. The least government, inhibitions, and encumbrances, the better the final human product.

Phillipe Pinel, William Tuke, and Benjamin Rush in the late 18th century and Dorothea Dix in the mid-19th strongly influenced the reformation of attitudes toward and treatment of society's deviants. Through their efforts, maladaptive, deviant behavior came to be thought of as a type of illness or disease. Pinel, Dix and others believed there was no difference between being "mentally ill" (or "crazy," as well as a dozen other epithets of the period) and having a broken leg. Instead of chaining people or burning them as witches, they believed these people should be put in general hospitals, state hospitals, or asylums.

8

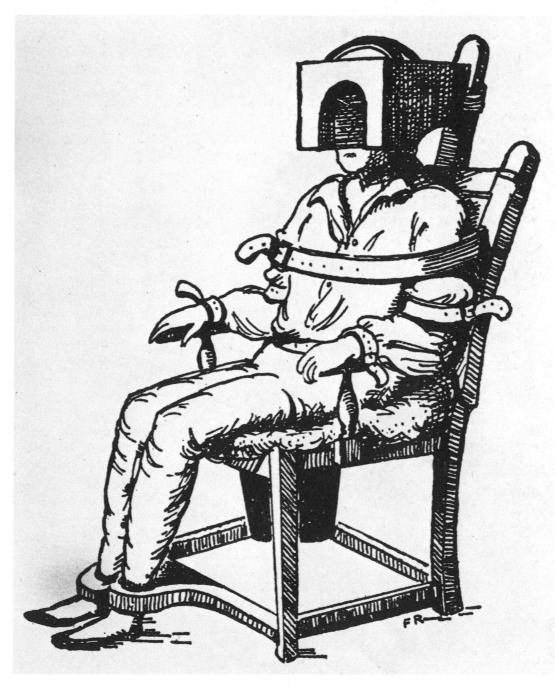

Benjamin Rush's "tranquilizing" chair, used to restrain unmanageable patients. (Courtesy The Bettmann Archive.)

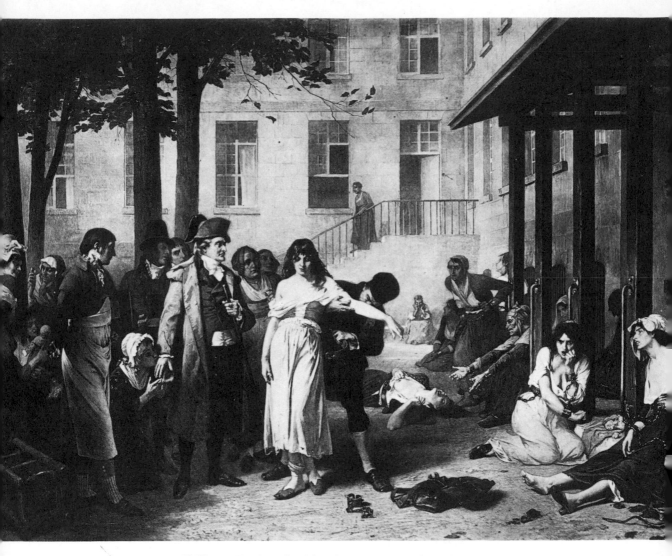

Phillippe Pinel unshackles the insane at Salpetrière in Paris, one of the milestones in psychiatric history. Painting by Robert T. Fleury. (Courtesy The Bettmann Archive.)

The Second Revolution or Wave

The second wave in the mental health revolution is usually attributed to Sigmund Freud, one of the great seminal thinkers of the 19th and 20th centuries. His many students and followers have played a major role in altering the mental health system, students such as Alfred Adler, Carl Jung, Wilhelm Stekel, and W. Reich.

Freud's theories and their ramifications have dominated the mental health field ever since. His towering stature has brought about a situation today which pretty much governs mental health delivery systems. Here are the prominent features of Freud's theories:

1. Deviant behavior is to be accepted as merely another form of physical illness. If a person acts in a deviant fashion, it is because of deep, unconscious forces which he is unable to control. These unconscious forces are the cause of his illness. They are comparable to such aspects of physical illness as fever, pain, swelling, or high blood pressure.

2. Inner events cause maladaptive behavior. If one wishes to treat the behavior, he must first explore the inner man for the cause or causes of the behavior, and the cause is usually a trauma that occurred during the first five years of a person's life.

3. The treatment to be provided is essentially the search for the inner cause of the behavior by means of *free association.* Free association is a technique in which the patient says everything that comes to mind, no matter what passes through his consciousness. Everything is to be openly and freely reported to the therapist. This process demanded complete trust by the patient and has been described as the royal road to the unconscious.

4. The therapist is a highly trained specialist (psychiatrist) who requires many years of preparation.

Although there are probably not more than 2,000 psychoanalysts in the entire United States, the Freudian approach dominates the mental health field. The method is clearly *intraorganismic;* that is, it focuses on an individual's inner happen-

11

ings. Nearly all treatment methods up to the present day have maintained this inner focus, and the service technologies are predicated on altering the inner man. It has become widely accepted that all deviant behavior results from an inner sickness. Psychiatrists have sought cures for mental illness just as others seek cures for cancer.

We refer to the position that has grown out of Freud's work as the *medical-Freudian-disease-cure-hospital-specialist model*, or *medical model* for short. (Details of the medical model are given in Part II.)

The Third Revolution or Wave

The third wave of the mental health revolution is still in its infancy, having begun since World War II. This revolution has had no one powerful thinker such as Freud behind it. It is a sort of grass roots movement. For an understanding of this revolution, the writings of the following thinkers will be helpful: Erwin Goffman [1961]; Gerald Caplan [1964]; Thomas Szasz [1961, 1970]; Walter Fisher, Joseph Mehr, and Philip Truckenbrod [1973a, 1973b, 1973c]; Maxwell Jones [1952]; A.H. Stanton and M.S. Schwartz [1954]; John and Elaine Cumming [1962]; Norris Hansell [1968]; Franklin Chu and S. Trotter [1962]; and B.F. Skinner [1971]. These writings are just a sample of the many forces coming together to produce a new movement.

The main focus of the human service movement and its revolutionary impact are given detail in Part IV. At this point, in order to provide some initial understanding of the problems of the human services and mental health, a number of our key themes are given:

1. There is less emphasis on evaluating and serving the inner man and more emphasis on evaluating and altering the social institutions that influence man's behavior. This orientation will be explained later in the book.

2. The human service model is based on the belief that the social system is both the cause of maladaptive behavior and the place to provide service. Examples of this service are: relink the patient to school, prepare him for a new occupation, link him to a cash economy, provide day care, create new institutions.

3. There is less emphasis on a causal past and more on the here

and now. One works with a patient in terms of where he is at the present and avoids deep probes into his past. This point can probably be best understood in terms of a case history. A woman in her late forties, for the first time in her life, begins to manifest behavior that might be described as psychotic or deviant: runs away from home, becomes terribly fearful, feels people are against her, attempts suicide, and develops the idea that she has a serious physical illness. Her family takes her to a psychoanalyst who diagnoses her condition as involutional psychosis with paranoid and depressive features (a change of life pattern). The patient is hospitalized in a well-known psychoanalytically oriented institution. The primary treatment is on the couch where the analyst probes her childhood. After several such hospitalizations and several analyses, the client is more distressed than ever and the family is desperate. The client is then taken to an institution of "last resort," the state hospital. The hospital staff, of course, does not have the resources for the deep probe. Instead they deal with the here and now. The facts are that this woman's children, in the pursuit of their careers, have gone off and abandoned her. This strange psychotic-form behavior has brought them back to her. The deviant behavior has been highly rewarded. The therapy involves confrontations, conscious decision making in maintaining a family network and the development of new attitudinal systems. Four or five years later our consumer still remains very much intact and we will never know what happened in those early years.

4. It is assumed that most maladaptive behavior does not result from a disease but is rather a matter of immediate life-space conditions. The patient is not a diseased person. His deviant behavior is viewed as a form of problem-solving when all other options have disappeared. The client in number 3 is not a diseased person. The human service worker would view her deviant behavior as a communication system, as a last-resort option when everything else has failed.

5. There are many different kinds of people, with diverse backgrounds, who can help the mental health patient. Most people in trouble turn to the family, good friends, and the clergy for help, and not to therapists. There will probably never be enough mental health workers to serve all of the mental health patients. The task of human service workers, therefore, is to identify those with the most potential for being helped.

6. This approach does not deny the usefulness of the medical model. However, the third revolution has introduced a new model, the *human service–social adaption–problem solving–behavioral––generalist–pragmatic model (human service model,* for short). This human service model has greatly extended the field; it complements the medical model and coexists in the same delivery system.

At first glance, there appears to be little difference between the medical and human service models, but in practice, they tend to guide mental health workers down very different roads. As noted above, the mental health worker who follows the guidelines of the medical model concentrates on the inner man. He attempts to understand a man's symbolic logic. He becomes a dedicated professional in a very private network. It is a gradual process which carries one further and further from everyday experience.

The human service worker, on the other hand, becomes increasingly involved with everyday events in the life of the patient who is trying to survive as a person. The worker becomes a pragmatic expediter. He becomes an expert in social institutions and social systems. He is not concerned with ideal solutions but rather seeks immediate answers to frustrations, obstacles, and difficulties. The preparation of the human service worker does not require elaborate schooling, whereas that of the medical model therapist does.

Why the Historical Perspective?

The presentation of this brief historical overview of the human service and mental health movement is to aid students in sorting out their thoughts. Although most mental health caregivers are not physicians, psychiatrists, or psychoanalysts, the medical model is the dominant orientation of our time. It appears that most new students entering the human service field develop this perspective. In fact, it is quite likely that an overwhelming majority of the people in the United States believe that maladaptive or deviant behavior is a result of an inner disease process which should be treated by a physician in or out of a hospital.

We want to provide a new perspective in this book; that is, we want to make other options available to the patient and the mental health care-giver. It is important that students, patients, and the interested public understand the medical model with all its limitations, which are related to the complexity of modern technology, the limited mental-health-patient population that can use this technology, and the high cost of services.

Before you can understand the human service model, you must put aside, if possible, any preconceived notions about the medical model. When a person acts in a deviant way, it is almost automatic to label that person as sick. It will be a major accomplishment for the reader to avoid this kind of thinking.

Detailed Listing of Goals, Objectives and Questions

As in any service book or clinical book, there are three large areas of development. First, there is the need to acquire a variety of information. Second, the student must become aware of the clinical technology and develop skills in using them. Third, one must have the necessary and appropriate attitudes in order to do the work required.

This last area—attitudes—is the most important in the mental health field. It is customary for agencies moving from the medical model to the human service model to encounter resistance from traditional professionals who think of themselves as white-collar workers specializing in patients' minds. The human service worker must work with the whole patient, including many of his unpleasant facets, for example, toilet training, cleanliness, eating habits, and rage. The attitudes necessary for functioning in the human service orientation are sometimes difficult to instill in those persons designated as professionals.

The list of goals, objectives, and questions this book raises are as follows:

1. You should understand contemporary mental health problems and issues as thoroughly as possible. An example of the mental health problem is expressed in the question: Are current, or traditional, mental health programs effective? This complicated question raises more questions: Is it possible to evaluate the existing models? Are human service programs evaluated? If we cannot or will not evaluate programs, why should they be supported? It is our belief

that this last question may be the key question—or problem—in the mental health field. There are other questions about the field that are nearly as important: Who should be institutionalized? Who should go to what institution? Who should make the decisions to send them to institutions? In what way are the various service agencies similar yet different? What exactly is mental illness? How do criminals differ from the mentally ill?

2. You should understand what constitutes maladaptation and deviancy in this society. Remember that there is no form of behavior that would be considered deviant *in all cultures in all historical periods.* If you examine the most atypical forms of behavior—incest, hallucinations, cannibalism, homicide, and patricide—you can find a culture which at some point in history considered that behavior acceptable and typical. Deviancy and maladaptation are defined differently at different times. Consider the following possibilities: mental illness is a myth; the concept of mental illness is useless; mental illness is used to make scapegoats of minorities and other "different" people.

3. As a corollary to number 2, there is the immediate and dramatic impact of a culture on an individual's way of living. The question of what constitutes deviancy shifts from generation to generation, and, since about 1960, even faster. In his writings, Freud described most of his clients as people who were overly inhibited and overly controlled. They were frequently diagnosed as hysterics, anxiety hysterics, or depressives—diagnoses that are rarely applied today. Today, patients are often at odds with society and are diagnosed as paranoids or sociopaths. They have lost their connection with friends and relatives. They are outside the normal boundaries of society. Atypical people today are at odds with their society. They are violent, exiled, at war, hostile; they are substituting inner chemical (drugs) experiences for human relationships. As one begins to grasp the relationship between culture and patterns of deviancy, a number of interesting questions occur: Should the maladjusted person be the client? Should the family be the client? Should society be the client? What should our service goal be? How does one properly identify mental health patients?

4. Number 3 raises the important question of which patients should receive priority. Should service-givers attend primarily to those seeking help who respond best to treatment? Or should they

treat only those who do not want help but who are still unable to function effectively in society? To a large extent, the answer will determine the nature of the service system.

5. One of our purposes in this book is to make you aware of cultural institutions and patterns and how they influence the development of the individual, and how they create maladaptive behavioral styles. You can better understand this if you first identify the basic needs of the individual in relation to his and his culture's attitudes toward these needs, as well as the institutions for serving the needs. We will discuss this later, with particular emphasis on Maslow's [1970] and Hansell's [1970] need models. Also see Table 1.1.

Table 1.1
Basic Needs in the Context of Their Cultural Institutions

Needs	Institutions
an intimate relationship	family and church
tie-in with cash economy	employer, family, public aid
link with peer group	school, church, social organizations
esteem (feeling of well-being)	family, employer, self, school, peer group
security	family, employer, intimate relationships

Behavioral styles, adaptive or maladaptive, grow out of society's reactions to the individual's needs. When these needs are denied or frustrated, the individual may turn to atypical (deviant) solutions.

6. Societies develop social institutions such as mental hospitals in order to cope with the maladaptive behavior of their citizens. In Table 1.2 are examples of deviancy and the institutions for dealing with it.

Table 1.2
Examples of Deviance and Relevant Societal Control Institutions

Example of Deviancy	Available Institution
voyeurism (peeping Tom)	mental hospital, prison, outpatient service
theft	police, prison, mental hospital
homicide	police, courts, prison, mental hospital
unable to support self	public aid, prison, mental hospital
mental retardation	special education, mental hospital
truancy	foster home, juvenile detention center

Many institutions have been created in American society to deal with deviance—mental hospitals, correctional institutions, police forces, public aid, special education, sheltered-care facilities, nursing homes, and private practitioners. You should be familiar with them and their function, resources, organizations, goals, staffing patterns, and so forth. This familiarity can come only from visits, work experiences, apprentice-work models, simulation experiences, and contact with people in the various agencies.

7. You should become familiar with the traditional mental health approach—the medical model—and this familiarity must begin with a historical perspective. Most social services come about for humanitarian reasons but continue for other reasons. Following are some themes of the medical model that should be understood:

A. You should be sensitive to the culture in which services are to be given. Mental health systems like most social systems are an expression of their culture. The individual is a microcosm of his culture and he internalizes its conflicts and solutions. A permissive society generates different conflicts and solutions to deviance than an authoritarian society.

B. You should be aware of the beliefs, assumptions, theories, and philosophy of the medical model.

C. Each model tends to generate its own system of delivery services. During the period in which the medical model was dominant, most mental health patients went to hospitals, clinics, or private practitioners. The model produces a pattern which is expressed in Table 1.3.

Table 1.3
Experience with Professional Help for Own Personal Problems
(From Elinson, Padilla, and Perkins [1967])

Did you ever go anywhere to get help for yourself for such a (mental or emotional) problem or condition?

Number quizzed, 2,118	total 100%
yes	8.6
no	91.1
No Answer	0.3

A. For all persons who ever had gone for help (N=183):

To what kinds of persons or places did you go?		Were you ever hospitalized for this condition?		Are you going anywhere for help now?	
	total 121.3%*		total 100.1%		total 100%
mental health professionals		yes	19.7	yes	16.9
psychiatrist	50.8	no	76.0	no	79.8
counselor	7.1	NA	4.4	NA	3.3
psychologist	14.8				
social worker	7.1				
other professionals or specialists					
physician	20.2				
clergyman	3.8				
lawyer	3.3				
other	14.2				

B. For all who are going for help now (N=31):
What kind of person are you seeing?

	total 103.1%*
mental health professionals	
psychiatrist	51.6
counselor	3.2
psychologist	12.9
social worker	3.2
other professionals or specialists	
physician	16.1
clergyman	3.2
other	12.9

*Percentages add to more than 100 because multiple answers were given.

D. Each model tends to generate its own technology. The medical model places considerable emphasis on technologies that attempt to describe and treat the inner man.

E. Each model tends to create professions that reflect the model. The medical model produces many specialists.

F. Each model tends to generate its own educational and service submodels. The medical model puts considerable emphasis on formal education.

G. The effectiveness of the medical model must be determined. So far, there has been little effort to do this. Headlines in our daily newspapers show *symptoms* of a failing mental health system.

8. Most universities still prepare their graduates within the

19

framework of the traditional medical model. These students are unprepared to work in today's service agencies and thus are largely ineffective. Once employed, they have to be reeducated before they are able to produce in a work situation.

9. Consider these questions: Who should deliver mental health services? Are the current systems for dealing with deviancy appropriate? How should mental health care-givers be educated? How should our resources be effectively used? Who should decide how mental health resources should be used? What is the role of the patient? What is the role of the interested public? Who should have the power to commit patients? What is the most effective service model?

10. Our goal in this book is to delineate the human service model, a model that can provide new fields of work and new careers. The human service model should be analyzed just as the traditional medical model was analyzed in number 7.

Summary

In this chapter we have set the stage for a discussion of the key issues in the field of mental health care. The service fields are going through major, revolutionary changes, which will crystallize in a new profession and a new field of activity. The change is probably best expressed in the rapid development of over 200 college programs in the area of human services: mental health, corrections, child care, mental retardation, law enforcement, and public aid. The human service model has emerged as a result of the shortcomings of the traditional service systems. It is not meant to replace the traditional systems, only to expand the various service fields.

Chapter 2 *Need-Motivational Models and Service Systems*

*I*n this chapter we will define the human service field and its relation to those patterns of behavior that are characterized as *mental health* or *mental illness*.

If you examine books on mental health, abnormal psychology, psychiatry, clinical psychology, and personality theory, you will see that there are a variety of approaches to understanding treatment and service. There have not, however, been any conceptual attempts to look at deviance and maladaptation in terms of the human service model.

The Need-Motivational Orientation

Our overall approach to human services and mental health in this book is based on a *need*, or *motivational*, model, a model which assumes that individuals (or all living creatures, for that matter) if they are to survive, must maintain their inner equilibrium or balance (homeostasis). A human being seeks what he needs and values most what he needs most.

sleeping infant ⟶ hunger drive ⟶ arousal of infant (stress of anxiety)

infant cries (signal system) ⟶ mothering person provides food
[human service worker]

hunger drive reduced ⟶ anxiety and stress reduced ⟶ infant returns to sleep
(homeostasis)

Figure 2.1. Homeostasis, or Seeking Balance in the Infant

Our modern concept of homeostasis (see Fig. 2.1) is based largely on the work of Walter B. Cannon [1932]. Homeostasis is the tendency of the body to maintain a balance of internal physiological conditions, balances which are necessary for the survival of an organism. For example, body temperature must not go too high or too low; blood pressure must not rise or fall beyond certain limits; the blood must not be too acidic or too alkaline. If a person's body gets too hot, he perspires and the evaporation of liquid cools the body. If the body gets too cold, he shivers and this steps up metabolism. Physiologists have discovered that many homeostatic mechanisms are involved in keeping conditions within normal limits. This process seems to be cyclical in nature (see Fig. 2.2).

MOTIVE

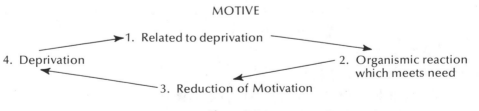

**Figure 2.2
Motivations Come and Go**

Ross Stagner [1948] has applied this physiological theory of motivation to other psychological drive states; it is a basic analog of motivation in this book. These psychological motives are given in Table 2.1

In serving the patient, therefore, it is vital that the service-giver grasp the patient's needs. Along with understanding the motivations of the patient, it is also essential to understand as much as possible the attitudes and values of the culture in which both the patient and service-giver live. In assessing an individual's needs, we should understand these values, as well as their possible effect on the patient. Every society has institutions to provide, modify, or reject the needs of its members, which is demonstrated in Table 1.2.

In short, people have needs which must be met. If the institutions that affect them interfere with or prevent the satisfaction of these needs, individuals may take on patterns of behavior that appear atypical, deviant, or abnormal to members of the community in general (see Tables 2.2, 2.3).

Need, or Motivational, Theories

There have been many theories of motivation in this century: Sigmund Freud [1920], Henry A. Murray [1938], Norris Hansell [1970], and Abraham Maslow [1970]. And there are several ways to identify these various needs: social approval, hostility, dependency, independence, achievement, security, attachment and affiliation, and the need for physical contact. For our purposes here, two major theories of motivation are important—Maslow's and Hansell's.

Abraham Maslow maintains that human beings have two distinct but interrelated types of needs, external and internal. His theoretical design postulates a hierarchy of needs which includes external and internal needs. Needs on the "lower" level are strongest as long as they are not fully satisfied. When they are satisfied, the "higher" needs become the primary focus; that is, one must meet the lower needs before he can attend to the higher ones. The hierarchy of needs is given in Figure 2.3.

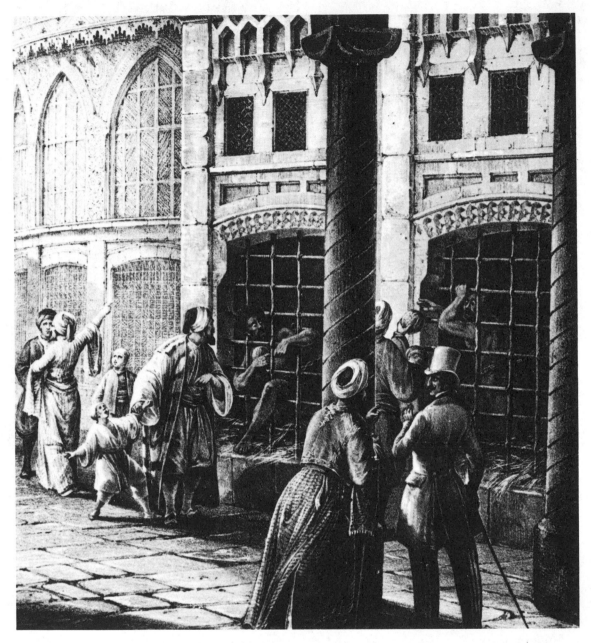

An early depiction of an asylum in Cairo, Egypt.
(Courtesy The Bettmann Archive.)

Table 2.1
A classification of major personal motives (after Murray, 1938)

Motive	Goal and effects
Abasement	To submit passively to others. To seek and accept injury, blame and criticism.
Achievement	To accomplish difficult tasks. To rival and surpass others.
Affiliation	To seek and enjoy cooperation with others. To make friends.
Aggression	To overcome opposition forcefully. To fight and revenge injury. To belittle, curse, or ridicule others.
Autonomy	To be free of restraints and obligations. To be independent and free to act according to impulse.
Counteraction	To master or make up for failure by renewed efforts. To overcome weakness and maintain pride and self-respect on a high level.
Deference	To admire and support a superior person. To yield eagerly to other people.
Defendence	To defend oneself against attack, criticism, or blame. To justify and vindicate oneself.
Dominance	To control and influence the behavior of others. To be a leader.
Exhibition	To make an impression. To be seen and heard by others. To show off.
Harmavoidance	To avoid pain, physical injury, illness, and death.
Infavoidance	To avoid humiliation. To refrain from action because of fear of failure.
Nurturance	To help and take care of sick or defenseless people. To assist others who are in trouble.
Order	To put things in order. To achieve cleanliness, arrangement, and organization.
Play	To devote one's free time to sports, games, and parties. To laugh and make a joke of everything. To be lighthearted and gay.
Rejection	To remain aloof and indifferent to an inferior person. To jilt or snub others.
Sentience	To seek and enjoy sensuous impressions and sensations. To genuinely enjoy the arts.

Figure 2.3 Maslow's Hierarchy of Needs

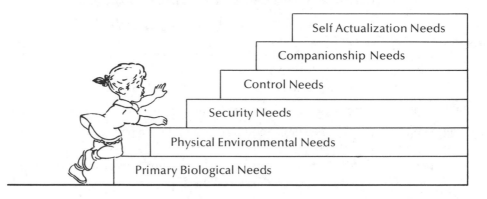

Level 1: *Primary biological needs*—food, sleep, waste elimination, breathing (basic life drives). This is an external motivation. By *external* we mean those motivations that are universal and common to the entire species. This is in contrast to the motivations that have to do with the individual.

Level 2: *Physical environmental needs*—shelter as a form of safety; familiar surroundings, a sense of home; reserves of food and water (future allocation); protective clothing, physical comfort, means of releasing drive energies (tension, anxiety, sexual). External motivation.

Level 3: *Security other than physical environmental security*—security of role and identity in the social system, security from knowledge of death (that is, religion), security from physical threat from other people, security from loss of personal property, security for controlling one's drives and other's drives not acceptable to the social system (morality). These needs are more internal.

Level 4: *Control needs*—manipulation of one's environment, taking risks for the purpose of emotional stimulation from risk-taking, wealth for the sake of importance (to control), physical force and social importance for the sake of control (the need to be strong). This is considered an internal need system.

Level 5: *Human companionship needs*—companionship and exchange of feeling, the desire for others to care and the desire to care for others, charity, hospitality, congeniality, social adaptation, and compromise for group harmony and a feeling of comradeship. Internal need system.

Level 6: *Self-actualization needs*—internal development and growth; to experience life; the need for happiness, autonomy and self-determination; communication with others for growth by exchange of ideas; to explore, innovate, synthesize, and create; to reach for higher potentials; to be introspective by understanding one's feelings and those of others, leading to intuition.

Table 2.2
Examples of Needs, Attitudes, and Solutions

Need	Possible Attitudes	Possible Solution
sex	Puritanical	marriage, celibacy
sex	permissive	promiscuity, prostitution, sex without marriage
sucking	nonpermissive, rigid	weaning at certain age
sucking	permissive	pacifier, child's decision
aggression	opposed to expression of aggression, rigid	force child to deny needs, block, set firm limits
aggression	permissive	encourage expression, allow play, competition

Table 2.3
Examples of Needs, Blocking Reactions, and Possible Deviance

Need	Cultural Blocking Reaction	Possible Deviance
sex	blocked, inhibited	exhibitionism, frigidity, impotence, voyeurism
aggression	blocked, inhibited	violence, extreme passivity
dependency	blocked, inhibited	overly dependent, antidependent
sucking	blocked, inhibited	drinking, smoking, obesity
achievement	blocked, inhibited	sense of failure, frustration, apathy

It is a basic element of Maslow's theory that a person moves up the hierarchy by meeting his needs at each level. Since people tend not to have all of what they need, once they have met a "level of needs," they move on to a "lower" ("higher" in hierarchy) priority need. (Note that Level 1 has the highest priority and Level 6 the lowest. This is because the "lower" levels are more closely related to survival and existence.) Obviously, without food and water, the individual will never get around to creativity and good interpersonal relations. As in all need-orientation models, it is the failure to meet needs that sets the stage for deviancy.

Hansell's motivational theory appears to be in accord with the human service orientation. He theorizes that individuals have to make seven basic attachments in order to meet their basic needs. If an individual does not make each attachment or adaptation, he goes into a crisis. First, the seven basic attachments:

1. The need to take in certain supplies—food, information, water. *Signs of failure:* boredom, physical malfunction, and loss of curiosity.

2. The need to maintain an intimate relationship—sex, someone to share secrets, a continuing relationship, a deep sense of closeness, and an exchange of deep feelings. *Signs of failure:* no reports of intimacy, lack of sexual contact, living alone, and minimal companionship.

3. The need to be part of a peer group—belong to a social club, church group, work group, social network, school group. *Signs of failure:* not feeling part of a group; seldom leaving the house; reporting the need for group contact; and feeling alone and isolated.

4. The need for a sense of identity—clarity of definitions, a sense of who one is, a cherishing of one's identity, the ability to make decisions. *Signs of failure:* ambiguity about oneself, decision-making difficulties, diffuseness of definitions, lack of clarity about self-boundaries.

5. The need for a social role that results in a sense of competency and esteem (feeling of well-being). *Signs of failure:* depression, sense of failure, no clear-cut work role, lack of dignity.

6. The need to be linked to a cash economy—have a job, be married to a person who supports his mate, be a member of a family,

be independently wealthy, receive Social Security benefits, be on public aid. *Signs of failure:* no purchasing power, not being able to purchase necessities.

7. The need for a comprehensive system of meaning—a system of priorities, the development of a methodology, or system, for making decisions. *Signs of failure:* no pattern to decision-making, drifting, unable to make choices within a priority system, and a sense of alienation from the mainstream of society.

According to Hansell's theory, you must make all seven attachments in order to meet the basic needs and avoid crisis and its consequent maladaptive behavior.

Setting the Stage: Crucial Questions

We will now consider the problems of the newborn child. He is a bundle of needs without any skills, mechanisms, or problem-solving abilities to meet these needs. Obviously, without a mother or mother substitute, the child would quickly perish. Motherhood and the family are the first institutions available for meeting the needs of the newborn child. In a sense, mother, father, and older siblings are the first human service workers the infant encounters.

At the other end of the spectrum, it is assumed that when an individual becomes an adult, he is able to identify and fulfill his needs. He begins to have problems when his expectations are not met and he goes into a crisis. This point is the essence of this book. The following questions will help define it:

What should be done for a person in crisis?
Who should serve him in crisis?
What resources should be made available to him in crisis?
How far should the care-giver go in meeting the needs of a person in crisis?
How much can be done for the person in crisis?

It is around these questions that the difference between two major models (the medical and the human service) revolves.

Below are several cases in which you are given an opportunity to

29

consider the appropriate services. After each case, there are two lists of services, one suggestive of the medical model and the other of the human service model.

1. In Chicago in 1972 there was a tragic train wreck in which many were killed, maimed, or traumatized. In such an event, one would expect serious interference with the survivors' ability to carry on their lives and meet their needs adequately. One would expect stress, crisis, maladaptations, and deviancy. How might mental health workers effectively help?

Medical Intervention
provide counseling; talk through grief; express anger about what
happened
provide group therapy sessions
diagnose emotional disturbances
hospitalize seriously upset persons
develop long-range therapy programs
Human Service Intervention
help provide persons with money
give aid to those who do not have hospitalization insurance
set up problem-solving sessions
help people find new jobs where necessary
help provide people with reputable legal services
function as advocate and expediter.

2. A man enters a state hospital in crisis—extremely anxious, hallucinating, distracted, unable to concentrate, confused. He had been forced to marry when he was 18 because he had made his girl friend pregnant. His family was angry and refused to help him. This incident had effectively blocked his plans for the future. He gave up his plan to go to college.

He took his new responsibility of being a husband and father seriously. He managed to get a job which at least allowed him to get by. In the next five years, his responsibilities and pains outran his income and satisfactions. Many times he thought of abandoning his family and simply disappearing. At the time of his hospitalization, his debts were out of control, he and his wife fought constantly, she

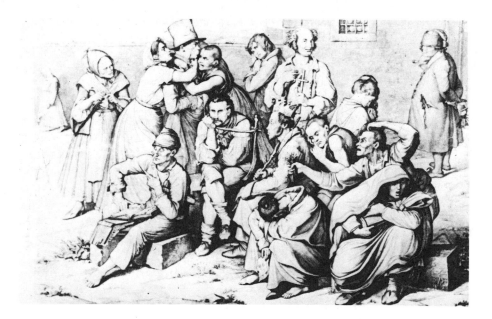

A contrast in the attempts to meet the needs of
presumably deviant individuals. Above, an old
engraving, *The Mad House* by Wilhelm V. Kaulbach; and
below, scenes in a school for retarded children today.
(Above, courtesy The Bettmann Archive; below, photo
by Costa Manos, Magnum.)

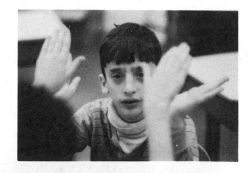

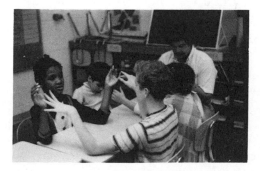

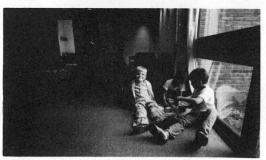

had rejected him sexually, and he had begun to suspect her of being unfaithful. Hospitalization appeared the only way out.

Medical Intervention
    diagnosis
    try to understand the underlying cause of the patient's problems
    explore his inner life through a psychotherapeutic procedure
    arrange a psychotherapeutic relationship as part of an aftercare
       program
Human Service Intervention
    arrange meetings with those important in the patient's life
    use the meetings to identify which of his basic needs are not being
       met
    develop a plan for meeting the needs, which is realistic and
       acceptable to him
    try to increase his problem-solving skills
    in this particular situation, focus on increasing his income and
       linking him to a more meaningful occupation

The Medical Model and the Need-Motivational Orientation

Next, we will consider the medical model in the context of Hansell's need theory and the role of care-givers in the model if the patient's needs are not being met. According to the medical model, a patient is brought (involuntarily) or brings himself (voluntarily) to a mental health care-giver; it is assumed that he is ill, that he has a disease. It is also assumed that the disease is the result of an inner process, an unmet and unknown inner motivation. The therapist tries to learn the causes and help the patient understand the cause through a process of discovery. This is known as insight. Once the patient is aware of the inner process (gains insight), he should have the personal resources to solve the problem; he should be able to identify his need, or needs, and take appropriate action to resolve them.

The traditional (medical) therapist takes a conservative part in this process. Generally, in this model, therapists are passive, non-directive, reflective; they are primarily listeners rather than doers.

They provide a minimum of material and practical aid. It is unlikely that they will intervene in the patient's practical problems such as lack of money, friends, sex, or education. The patient is informed that these are problems he must learn to solve.

There are many patients who benefit from this approach but it is not and can not be universally effective. It requires a certain amount of time (usually years), a good deal money (usually $40 a session), a certain amount of education, and an insightful type mind.

By using the human service model, we have redefined the role of the mental health care-giver in treating a patient. Instead of passive, conservative workers, we have activists, interventionists, doers, and risk-takers. In the human service model, if the patient does not have enough money, the human services worker may link him to a welfare system or help him find a job. If the patient finds it difficult to join a social organization, the worker may try to create a new social organization. The human service worker is an expediter, facilitator, ombudsman, friend, depending on what is needed.

This change in orientation has resulted in a much greater number of people who can be helped. Those who before didn't have the personal resources (financial, intellectual, communication skills, motivation) to use and gain from the medical model, have become eligible for human services.

In the human service model, mental health workers participate in all phases of need-satisfaction. They do not limit themselves to a specific psychotherapeutic technology or process such as insight. If you consider this model in the context of Hansell's seven attachments, you must think of the human service worker as one who will do everything necessary to maintain or restore the seven attachments.

Summary

We have analyzed the human service orientation in this chapter. The orientation is not a tight operational one; rather, it is a *sense of definition*. The human service model can best be understood in the context of a need, or motivational, theory. An individual's deviancy is attributed to his inability to meet his needs appropriately. Service-givers disagree as to how much the service-giver should participate in trying to meet the needs of the patient. It is this difference in attitude that distinguishes the human service worker from the traditional (medical) worker.

Chapter 3 *Issues, Problems, and Questions in Human Services and Mental Health*

*I*n Chapter 2, the authors introduced a major concept or theme of the book—the need or motivational orientation to understanding the human service model and deviancy. It is important to understand that when the vital needs of an individual are impeded or blocked, it will typically result in deviant or maladaptive behavior. It is around the task of how to aid the client that the medical and human service models differ in defining their tasks.

Those who use the medical model typically have defined their task as helping the patient sort out and identify his needs through therapy—insight, free association, interpretation, projective techniques, reflection, and chemotherapy. Once the patient has been aided in this process, it is his responsibility to take the necessary steps to meet these needs. The therapist in this system seldom leaves his office.

The human service model greatly *expands* the role of the therapist or service-giver. They not only actively aid the client in sorting out and identifying his needs, but these workers also function as expeditors, facilitators, ombudsmen, helpers, and advocates in aiding the client provide for these needs. The human service workers not only function in offices, but they also go out into the streets and aid the client in the process of survival.

The differences between the two models raise a variety of issues, problems, and questions. In this chapter our task is to identify and clarify them. This will aid readers to sort out and categorize the primary themes of the book. This sorting out will begin by discussing the major issues and problems.

Specificity and Nonspecificity

Although the issue of specificity versus nonspecificity emerges from the need-motivational model, it rivals that concept in importance insofar as determining work patterns and workloads of mental health service-givers. Let us first define the issue. It begins with the assumption of the need-motivational model, that deviancy results from unmet needs. If this is so, there are two basic theoretical questions: How specific does one have to be in identifying the unmet need? How specific must a treatment method be in providing the service, or object, in meeting the need?

We can clarify this with an example from physical medicine. A mother wakes up one morning to find her baby sick with a high fever, loss of appetite, and discomfort. She immediately calls her pediatrician. On the phone the pediatrician is unable to diagnose the illness or identify the cause. He takes a *nonspecific* approach. He prescribes a wide-spectrum antibiotic for a variety of infections. If after a prescribed period of time, the child does not improve, the pediatrician will have the mother bring the child in for a more specific examination. The second step is not always required, since much of the time, the nonspecific orientation eliminates the infection.

In the medical model the treatment typically has been *specific*. Freud [1920] designed a therapeutic process in which one sorts out and identifies with the clients the specific dominant need (the basic wish) of the client. This is a complicated and lengthy process, which requires a highly trained therapist. The therapy, or *medicine*, of the system must be *prescriptively specific* to the needs of the patient.

An Example of the Medical Model

A female patient comes to an analyst with a variety of symptoms, including anxiety, physical pains, and general unhappiness. In effect, an understanding is reached between the patient and therapist, which will include the fee, pattern of meetings (frequency, length of session), obligations of each, etc.

It is an assumption of the model that the client's problems stem from incidents that occurred early in her life (the first five years). That is, the patient as a child was rejected by the parents at some point in her development because of the parents' inadequacies. She, in turn, *returned to her last childhood point of satisfaction* and organized her life around this motivational system. It is the task of the therapist to help the patient return to this period and in meticulous detail reconstruct the past events. It is part of the theory of this model that, as the patient understands what took place between her and each of her parents, she will initiate a process of restructuring her life, and there will be an alteration of the motivational system. But she must understand exactly her mother's and father's roles in regard to her and to each other, as well as the patterns of dependency, hostility, and sexuality as they existed in that household. This is a lengthy process; it usually takes a minimum of two years.

Proponents of the human service model agree that there are times in which it is vital that the human service worker understand the individual in some detail. But they suggest that this is the exception and not the rule, feeling that with limited resources (therapists, clinics, time, money), one can be more effective using a wide-spectrum approach.

An Example of the Human Service Model

Suppose a hundred people arrive for mental health services because they are unable to support themselves. There may be many reasons why they have these problems, but if an attempt is made to analyze each of them, seeking out the childhood fixations that caused the problems, the search will become almost endless and enorm-

37

ously costly. The general human service approach would be to relink them economically to society: jobs, reeducation, and public aid if necessary. It would certainly not be anticipated that all 100 people would be served effectively on the way. For the remainder, there would be other nonspecific solutions. Perhaps for a few, the human service worker might pursue a specific therapy.

The specific-nonspecific issue is important in defining the work roles of mental health care-givers. We will return to this issue throughout the book.

Target Population

Who is to be served? It appears that our two models lead toward different target populations. Specifically, if you examine the medical model in regard to its need-motivation orientation and its emphasis on specificity, compared to the need-motivational orientation and nonspecificity emphasis of the human service orientation, you end up with something very different.

The medical model requires the patient to understand his problems *specifically* and with the insight gained, take the necessary action to solve his problems. This model seems to require a high-resource person—good intelligence, sophisticated at problem-solving, articulate, with average or above income. Generally, it has been a model designed for middle-class people of above-average intelligence.

The human service model has been designed particularly to meet the person *wherever he is.* Anyone who is maladaptive because of his inability to meet his needs is theoretically eligible for service. We are referring to a cafeteria of services—talking, linking, expediting, helping, and facilitating. It is a recognition of the great importance that an individual must meet his needs.

Boundaries

It should be clear by now that the boundaries of the field are not precise. They appear to depend largely on the model used. In the traditional medical model there are clearer boundaries. Workers in this field infer that maladaptive behavior is the result of a disease and the disease be treated by a medical person according to a medical methodology; that is, we identify the disease (diagnosis) and treat the patient.

In the last 10 or 15 years, coincident with the emergence of the human service model, the boundaries have become vague and imprecise. A much larger target population is being served. In the spirit of the human service model, many new services are being provided through the development of new delivery systems and technologies. In fact, there appears to be a new consumerism which is no longer satisfied with the old mental health boundaries. We are being forced to reconsider the entire mental health system.

It should be pointed out that the expanding boundaries of mental health are also forcing mental health workers to reconsider the relationship of mental health to other human service agencies. Who should be placed in prison? Who should be placed in a mental hospital? Who should have the responsibility for public aid? What should the relationship between police departments and mental health workers be? In short, the boundaries between agencies are nowhere near being precise. For all who suffer from maladaptive behavior, the initial relationship probably should be through a generalist human service worker, with specialist departments being brought in only when the human service approach has proven ineffective. (This is explored in Part IV.)

Since there is a continuous comparison between the medical and human service models in this book, it is important to consider two vital issues—program evaluation and power struggles.

Program Evaluation

Recently the authors of this book completed a book entitled *Power, Greed, and Stupidity in the Mental Health Racket* [1973]. The title was chosen to point up our belief that there has not been and is not now an acceptable, objective, scientific procedure for evaluating the effectiveness of mental health programs. Without such a procedure, most decisions will be made on the basis of *power, greed, and stupidity.* Failure to evaluate *at all* is typical not only of the mental health field but of almost all human service agencies—universities, correctional institutions, retardation centers, public aid, elementary schools, and so on.

There have been many attempts to make meaningful evaluations—Mowrer [1953], Fiedler [1951], McQuitty [1938], Eysenck [1966]—yet there has been no large mental health organization such as a Department of Mental Health for developing a workable evaluation procedure that could be the basis of a decision-making process. Some examples of what can happen without such a procedure follow.

Open-ended Psychotherapy

A person enters psychotherapy with a specific symptom or problem. After 10 sessions the symptom disappears. Does the patient stop therapy at this time? The answer is usually no, because neither he nor the therapist can predict with precision whether the problem has disappeared or the symptom has merely changed. There does not seem to be an easy solution as to when a patient separates from psychotherapy. There is no meaningful information as to when the effects from psychotherapy have been maximized. Psychotherapy can last one session or go on endlessly, and there is no scientific evidence to indicate whether the endless therapy has been more effective than the one session.

A State Governor

A governor takes office at a time when the state Department of Mental Health is seriously disorganized. He appoints a creative and clever director who in a period of eight years brings meaningful organization and growth to the department. On any given day, the department may appear dehumanizing, even brutal, but in terms of additional staff, reduced patient load, and remodeling of residential facilities, the director has accomplished a minor miracle.

There is an election and a governor from another party is elected. The incoming governor claims that the Department of Mental Health is in wretched shape; he fires the director and replaces him with a new director who begins to move the department in another direction. Without an effective evaluation program it is difficult to take a position in opposition to a new political force. This situation occurs at almost every election in which there is a shift in political parties.

It is even more important today, when there are at least two major mental health models in conflict, to have an objective procedure for measuring program effectiveness. As was pointed out in Chapter 2, it is important to know how far to go in helping mental health patients meet their needs. There is potential for a meaningful experiment with the two models. One thing is certain: if there is no resolution of the problem of measuring program effectiveness through objective scientific procedures, politics and power will become the ultimate criteria for decision making.

Power Struggles in the Mental Health Field

Anyone who has worked in a large human service agency has experienced the endless power struggles that take place in them. Even though there are daily examples of these struggles, many human service workers are unaware of or deny that they take place. They, as well as administrators, prefer to believe that service agency operations are devoted to humanitarianism, altruism, love, dedication, and good will. Unfortunately, this is not always true. Mental health services in the United States are a multibillion-dollar industry and those in control have a great deal to protect.

From Freud to the present, medical people have controlled the field of mental health. In most governmental agencies relating to mental health, the important posts are held by medical persons, for example, directors of departments of mental health, superintendents, and directors of mental health units in the armed forces. The power struggles in the field are not significantly different from those occurring within or between various industrial systems. The historical wave we call the Third Revolution has the possibility of a major shift in the power patterns within the mental health field.

The Human Service Profession

An agency has about 300 people who come to it each month seeking help. The workers at the "front door" describe the needs of these people as *human service* needs; that is, many of their *people needs* are not being met. They lack money, education, family, friends,

41

sex, and most other human resources. Their problems do not seem to be the result of diseases. It is the staff's opinion that most of them don't require medical services or hospitals but rather jobs, housing, sex partners, and money. If one follows this line of thought far enough, it becomes apparent that our society needs fewer hospitals and less medical services, that a new mainstream profession is needed: the human service profession.

Obviously such a movement will encounter resistance from the medical Establishment. It is only human nature for entrenched power groups to want to hold onto their power. There seems to be no question that the revolution occurring in the field of mental health is bringing the struggle to a head. The reader should be sensitive to this struggle and be aware of the rational and irrational forces that go into decision-making in the mental health field.

Up to now in this book, we have presented these main issues and problems:

The two major, mental health models
The need-motivational models
Different motivational models
The possible cause of deviancy
Focusing on and treating the inner man
Specificity and nonspecificity
Target populations
Boundaries
Evaluation
Power struggles

In the remainder of this chapter, we will set forth questions and explanations of questions stemming from these issues and problems, which, it is hoped, will further your understanding of the many problems involved.

Is there such a condition that we can legitimately call mental illness? It would be useful for you to read Thomas Szasz [1961], Ronald Leifer [1969], and Fisher, Mehr, and Truckenbrod [1973] for a deeper understanding of this issue. Essentially, the question being asked is whether the deviant behavior of some persons can best be explained in terms of a sickness or disease. That is, are some forms of deviancy an expression of an inner neurological or biochemical disorder

Frank Leslie's Popular Monthly

Vol. XIV.—No. 5.   NOVEMBER, 1882. $3.00 Per Annum.

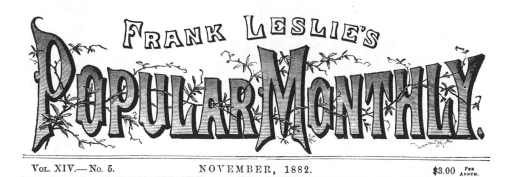

HOW TO DECIDE THAT A MAN IS INSANE, AND HOW TO TREAT HIM IF HE IS.

Ever since the immortal author of "Don Quixote" presented a type of mental aberration, in which natural shrewdness and sound sense blended with the craziest ideas drawn from fiction, the borderland between reason and insanity has been a subject of study.

Cervantes wrote after witnessing many cases of insanity, and the delineation of the gentleman of La Mancha shows the result of examination.

Insanity is very deceptive. It seems to sharpen natural shrewdness and cunning, so that at times it will puzzle the most expert practitioner. The wife of a member of Parliament sent once most urgently for a famous London physician. He responded, but soon after being announced was met in the drawing-room by the gentleman himself, who expressed his gratification on his timely call. He had been about to summon him, for he was extremely anxious about his wife. He was convinced that she was becoming mentally unsound, and wished the physician's opinion in regard to her, and the best treatment to be adopted. He was calm, clear and able, as he had shown himself on the floor of the House of Commons. He left the room to send his wife to the drawing-room. She entered in a few minutes, flying rather than walking, her attire disordered, her eyes bloodshot, her whole person showing extraordinary excitement, and a neglect of all that care for personal appearance that seems inherent in a lady. In somewhat disconnected phrases she began to tell her trouble. Her husband, gifted, talented, was evidently from overwork becoming insane. She began to describe his acts showing an unbalanced mind. The physician was astounded. Each asserted the other to be insane. To all appearance the calm, dignified husband was in full

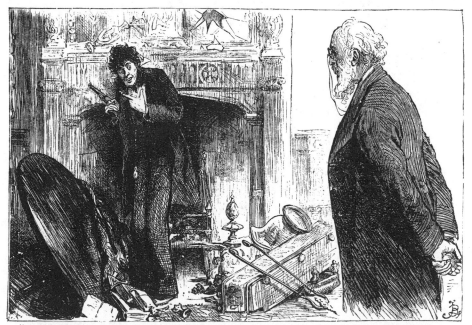

"THE HUSBAND, IN A PAROXYSM OF MANIA, STANDING IN THE WRECKED DRAWING-ROOM, STILL HOLDING A PISTOL WHICH HE HAD DISCHARGED AT AN IMAGINARY FOE IN THE MANTEL MIRROR."

Vol. XIV., No. 5—33.

A page from a magazine article in 1882, describing how to evaluate whether a person was insane. (Courtesy The Bettmann Archive.)

which *parallels* more traditional forms of sickness such as measles, chicken pox, or cancer? It does seem probable that metabolic disturbances can cause bizarre behavior.

Are there a number of different factors which may cause deviant behavior? Is it possible that deviant behavior is caused by a variety of factors—biochemical, neurological, childhood experiences, an unpleasant life pattern, heredity? In the literature on the subject are a number of mental health experts who take different positions: Freud [1920], Rogers [1942], Sarbin [1964], Kolb [1968].

Do all persons requiring mental health services require the same kind of treatment? Apparently, since there are a variety of factors that contribute to maladaptive behavior, mental health workers require an assortment of treatments in order to serve their patients. If one becomes emotionally disturbed because he is unable to master his everyday problems, should he be treated as someone who is malfunctioning because of a neurological disorder?

What kinds of problems bring a patient to a mental health worker? This is obviously an important issue. It would seem that how one answers the question could determine the appropriate model to use. If patients are truly sick in the traditional sense, care-givers should be prepared to use the medical model. On the other hand, if the problems that bring the patient to the mental health care-giver are related to human services issues, care-givers must provide an alternative to the medical model.

How far should human service workers go in meeting patients' needs? Obviously some service-givers feel the workers should merely talk with the patient and help him sort out his problems. This is in contrast to those mental health care-givers who suggest doing everything necessary to meet the needs of the client. If service-givers maximize their service to the patient, do they risk making the patient *permanently* dependent on them?

Are human service workers more effective in serving patients when their primary focus is on altering the environment of the individual? The human service model is oriented toward the environment rather than the inner man (unconscious). It assumes that behavior is more a

44

function of an individual's immediate situation and the external pressures on him. Some believe that treatment based on this orientation works more quickly and more effectively: Lewin [1935], Skinner [1938], and Fisher, Mehr, and Truckenbrod [1973a, 1973b, 1973c].

Who is prepared to serve the patient? Some have recommended that the mental health care-giver be a highly educated and trained therapist. This is obviously in the tradition of medicine, where physicians are trained for many years in highly sophisticated techniques and equipment. For instance, it takes a minimum of 14 years beyond high school to become a certified psychiatrist.

There is an opposing position which places minimum stress on schooling and credentials. In the human service model, it is held that the personal equation is the crucial factor in providing services, that is, a person's appearance, personality, temperament, general intelligence, and other personal characteristics, are more important than formal schooling.

What special skills should a mental health worker have? Although there has been some kind of training for mental health workers for 200 years, there has never been objectively-identified skills which it can be assumed are necessary in order to provide effective mental health services. There is the paradox of educating thousands of people in the field without developing a meaningful methodology for identifying the competencies.

Is there a need for trained therapists? Basically this question asks: is therapy an experience which only *trained* therapists can deliver? If you think of serving the deviant person in terms of meeting his unmet needs, can you then deny the therapeutic role to anyone who participates in this process? Is everybody a therapist? Is no one? Can we say that there is *therapy* but there are no *therapists?*

What changes can service-givers bring about in the patient? This is a basic question. If care-givers cannot substantiate the belief that they can bring about major and meaningful changes in the makeup of an individual, it is absurd to continue him in lengthy, complicated therapy. Somehow therapy must be tailored to what is *achievable* and *probable.*

45

Summary

In this chapter we have attempted to identify many of the crucial issues, themes, and problems in the human service and mental health fields. The task at this point in the book is not to provide answers, but to sensitize the reader to the issues.

Chapter 4 *Mental Health Consumers and New Public Health Techniques*

The Little Boy

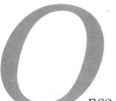nce a little boy lived in a large city with his mother and father. One day the boy's mother took him to a psychoanalyst. The boy's mother waited outside while the boy went into the analyst's office. The office was dim and had many books and a big chair and couch. The analyst asked the boy if he wanted to come to see him. But the boy didn't say anything and just looked at the analyst. The analyst smoked his pipe and looked back at the boy.

Every day after that, the boy went to see the analyst. They both sat there, the analyst in his big chair, the boy on the couch. They would look at each other and the analyst would smoke his pipe. Sometimes he would say something to the boy. Once he said that the boy must be very frightened, that if he were the boy, he would be frightened too. But the boy didn't say anything. Another time the analyst said that the boy must be very angry to have to come to the analyst's office every day. But the boy only looked at the analyst and said nothing.

Sometimes at home, the boy's father asked him what went on at the analyst's office. He asked the boy if he said anything to the analyst or if he had learned anything from him. But the boy didn't say anything.

Time passed—months, then years. Every day except weekends the boy went to the analyst's office. They just sat there. The analyst smoked his pipe and sometimes said something. The boy merely sat and looked at the analyst and said nothing.

One day after many years, the boy spoke. He told the analyst that he had decided long ago never to speak to anyone ever and that he was telling the analyst this because he thought the analyst was a nice man.

The analyst wept. But the little boy never spoke to anyone again. (B. Green [1973])

What were your feelings when you finished reading this story? Is it a study in absurdity? Is the analyst a silly, impotent man? Is being a "nice man" sufficient? Should the boy have been forced to talk? Would it have been best to ignore his silence?

You might well think about these questions and any others that come to mind. Also, it may be interesting at the conclusion of this book to return to this story and reconsider the questions and your answers.

An Overnight Change

The next story involves the kind of services that should be made available to mental health patients.

In the mid-fifties one of the authors of this book, at the request of a psychology intern, undertook the treatment of a patient who was variously diagnosed Schizophrenic Reaction hebephrenic type and Schizophrenic Reaction, chronic undifferentiated type. In other words, he was considered very "crazy." The intern wanted to observe treatment in progress, to participate in the process; but at the same time, he didn't want to harm the patient or feel that he would be wasting the patient's time.

A patient was picked out who had been in the institution nine years and was now in a "back ward." At the time, the hospital was

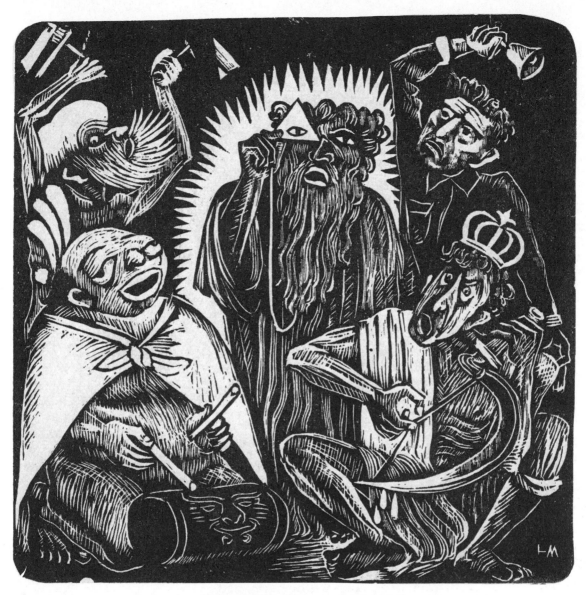

Woodcut by L. Mendez, *The Insane* (1932). (Courtesy
New York Public Library.)

organized around a system of isolating patients to progressively worse wards as their competency declined. This particular patient had reached the bottom of the system. He was selected primarily because prior to hospitalization he had shown certain developed resources such as being a good musician and attending college for several years.

At first there seemed no hope of intervening effectively. The patient was a classic example of the *alleged process* schizophrenic; the *opening phase* of his illness resembled catatonia, which was followed by a regression to paranoid patterns (building his own world) and then a decline in behavior which was labeled hebe-phrenic (a kind of anarchy). The therapists would like to have helped him, but there seemed little chance of doing so. The patient had a grave prognosis.

In terms of their feelings about the case, the therapists' other obligations, and reservations about spending time with the patient, it was arranged so that we saw him twice a week in one-hour sessions in the offices of the senior therapist. The therapeutic approach was modeled on the various dyadic systems extant at the time: Rogers [1961], Freud [1920], Adler [1924], and others. The therapists were to be primarily listeners; the patient was to recognize his illness and accept responsibility for it; the therapists were to achieve communication with the unconscious systems and modify them if possible. The patient did not understand the approach, nor did he choose to participate in it.

Before discussing the therapeutic approach further, let us look at some of the patient's characteristics:

1. He was uninhibited; he constantly and publicly masturbated.
2. He tolerated no tension and passed gas at the slightest provocation.
3. He urinated wherever he happened to be.
4. He delighted in his hallucinations.
5. He was unconcerned about wearing clothes.
6. He had a massive greed, devouring everything in sight.

At first the patient attended the therapy sessions without much coaxing, but once in the sessions, he refused to participate. This was the classic "irreversible schizophrenic." Without good cause, the two therapists kept at it even when it seemed wise to discontinue the therapy. The patient became bored with his role and refused to come to the sessions. The two therapists, disregarding their past training, which indicated that a patient should be well motivated, forced the patient to attend the sessions. In the months that followed, there were attempts by the patient to set a fire in the therapists' office; he urinated in inappropriate places; he frequently had to be physically restrained. Therapy became a structuring, limiting, restraining procedure.

After several effort-filled months in which therapy was moved out of the office onto the grounds, at the piano and into various activities, the entire experience reached a super blow-up. The patient, by all accounts, seemed to be totally crazy—screaming, running, jumping, and rolling. When this came to an end through appropriate limits to his behavior through external controls, he appeared to make a complete turnaround. It was a day-and-night experience. He seemed to *capitulate* and actually apologized for behaving as he had for the past nine years. Within a short time, he left the hospital. Unfortunately (or fortunately), we never followed up on him, nor have we heard from him since.

A Changing Orientation

The move to this activist type of service orientation was not original or unique to the therapists or to the agency. John Rosen [1952] has reported similar experiences. There are several key themes involved in this approach which are different from the dominant medical model of the 1950s:

The therapist does not seek out the causal elements of the past. Therapy focuses on the here-and-now relationship between the patient and the therapist.

In encountering the patient, the therapist forces him to use his own decision-making apparatus to change his behavior. The patient is held responsible for his behavior.

The therapist becomes more directly involved with the patient, including physical restraint and forcing the patient to clean up the messes he makes (restitutional therapy).

The therapist functions more out of a family model than a hospital model. He is involved in the process of socializing the patient.

51

The therapist becomes involved with all of the patient's needs and participates more actively in meeting these needs.

After 10 years of observing this approach in one-to-one service relationships, the senior therapist and several psychology interns used the same methodology in a group setting.

A "Snake Pit" Group

Three psychology interns asked the senior therapist if he would participate in a group with them in order to provide them with a learning experience. The therapists talked about the case and thought it might be interesting to try to pursue the same pattern on a group basis. The senior therapist was responsible for the extended-care service in his agency. *Extended-care* patients were those between 18 and 60 who had been hospitalized over 90 days.

After considerable discussion it was decided to set up a group of patients. We asked the team leaders in the extended-care service to provide us with five of their most bizarre, regressed, and disturbed patients. We actually worked with eight patients but no more than five at one time. The patients had the following general characteristics:

They were generally in their forties, with the exception of one man in his middle twenties.

They were of both sexes.

They had spent most of their adult lives in mental institutions.

They were all diagnosed as schizophrenic and were considered to have a grave prognosis.

They all demonstrated bizarre and regressed behavior—poor toilet control, odd language usage, strange dress, poor controls, strange eating habits.

All rejected authority and structure.

The four therapists decided that during the first session they would evaluate the situation, with a minimum of structuring. This session was like the classical "snake pit." The patients were allowed complete freedom, except that they could not leave the room. They wet the floor and themselves. They babbled incoherently. They wan-

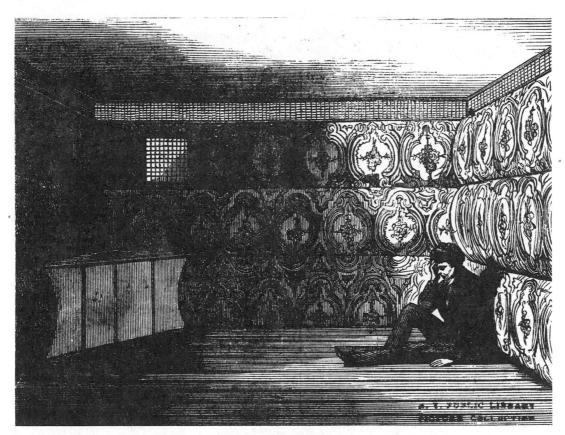

Early examples of the treatment of mental patients. Above, a 19th-century padded cell; below, use of the straitjacket, front and back, and use of belt and shackles. (Above, courtesy New York Public Library; below, courtesy The Bettmann Archive.)

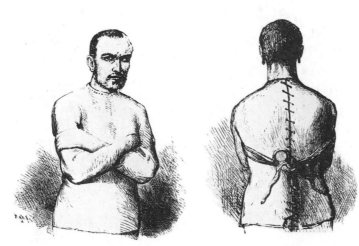

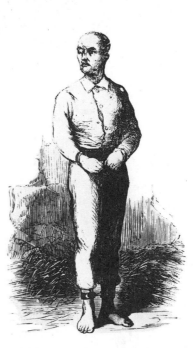

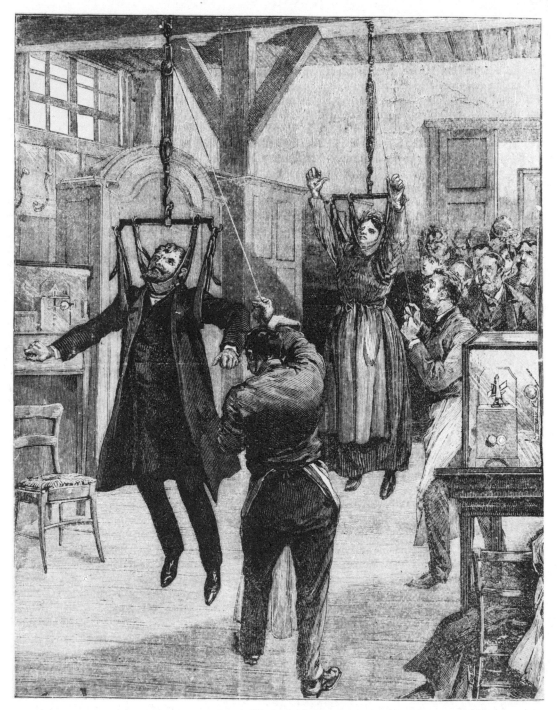

Suspensory treatment for atoxia in an old-time asylum.
(Courtesy The Bettmann Archive.)

dered aimlessly around the room. They assumed strange postures. It was chaos, anarchy, and absurdity.

A therapeutic strategy was prepared for the next session, which was explained to the patients:

1. The patients were told that they would not assume responsibility for themselves; for the time being, the therapists would make the decisions.

2. If and when they assumed responsibility, they could participate in the decision-making.

3. The group would continue for 10 one-hour sessions, with one session per week.

4. The patients would be required to come.

5. During these sessions they would not be allowed to behave bizarrely (the therapists explained what they meant by *bizarre*: wetting of self or floor, wandering around the room, physical attacks, unintelligible talk, and leaving the room).

6. The therapists explained what would happen if the patients did not follow the rules: if they wet the floor, they would have to clean it up; if they physically attacked someone, or did not remain in their chair, they would be restrained; certain ward privileges would be withdrawn if they did not cooperate.

7. "Craziness" simply would not be tolerated.

A modest goal was set for the group: the ending of bizarre behavior. Stabilization of their behavior, discharge from the hospital, improved reorganization of their lives would be bonuses.

The next session went as expected. The patients tried to continue their bizarre behavior while the therapists mobilized to discourage the attempt. It was a struggle between the socializers and the unsocialized. But after two sessions the behavior disappeared. No one wet the floor, the violence disappeared, the patients talked coherently, their appearance markedly improved, and communication was verbal rather than behavioral. After 10 sessions the group appeared to be functioning much as any societal group in a group therapy session.

There were some bonuses—several began the process of reintegration, and several were discharged. Since then, a new agency program has been developed around this model. The key theme of this group therapy methodology was *massive intervention of the*

55

therapists. The role of the care-giver is far different and more intrusive than that of the therapist using the traditional technique.

We now present some unusual cases, which can be thought of as *confrontation* or *existential experiences* (life versus death events) and which have vital implications for mental health service-givers.

Cancer as an Antidote

The patient was a 57-year-old-woman who had been in state residential facilities since she was 15, when in the eyes of her family, she had begun to act strangely. She had been a good student until then, and in nearly every way was the parent's ideal of a perfect child: she helped her mother in the house, was obedient and courteous; she dressed nicely but did not date. Suddenly she became unraveled, as if someone had grabbed a loose thread. All of the "goods" were replaced by "bads." The parents took her to their family doctor who referred them to a private hospital. Finally they reached the ultimate solution—the state hospital.

After about five years, everyone gave up. Then the girl, now 20, was placed in a "ward of no return" where she spent the next 37 years—in her own excrement, her own world, with total disregard for anyone or anything. During these years she was subjected to various therapies—insulin shock, electric shock, barbiturates, hydrotherapy, packs, and tranquilizers—all to no avail. She was never *cured*.

About six months before her 57th birthday, she became physically ill. The illness was diagnosed as terminal cancer. As she neared death, her long-time psychiatric symptoms seemed to melt away, and for the last month of her life she was rational and realistic by most standards. Other cases similar to this one have been reported in other state hospitals, which leads us to the hypothesis that possible extreme deviance cannot be maintained in times of great realistic stress. Existential crises may be antidotes for withdrawal.

War and Hospitals

This is an account of a mental hospital in a London suburb, which was the British equivalent of a state hospital, during the heavy bombing raids by the Germans in World War II. In a large raid several bombers overshot London and instead bombed the suburb where the hospital was, shattering windows and blowing the doors off their hinges. The staff of the hospital were pressed into service to aid the areas most heavily hit, which left the patients temporarily without a staff to care for them. Left to their own devices and resources, the patients organized work crews and cleaned up the debris. They worked at repairing the damage and temporarily lived in the hospital as a community group. There were no suicides, homicides, or escapes.

From such experiences new variables in service emerged. Care-givers now had to think about the importance of expectations and environmental settings as influences on altering a patient's be-havior. These ideas were explored more fully after the war and led to new philosophies and ideologies in treatment. Maxwell Jones [1952] reports that this knowledge was the beginning of the patient-government movement. More on this later in the chapter.

An Existential Crisis

In a journal article, LeGuillant [1946-47] described what hap-pened at a French mental hospital in France during World War II. The hospital lay in the path of the German army. Most of the patients had been sent home to their relatives, but 153 who were considered too ill to travel were to be escorted to safety by the hospital staff. But the Germans moved faster than anticipated, and the patients were on their own.

The story ends here until after the war, when a commission was set up to find out what had become of the patients. Most were traced; of them, 56 (37%) were found to have made appropriate community adjustments. *Hopeless* patients had been placed in an existential crisis encumbered with responsibility for themselves and were forced to make decisions. They far exceeded the expectations of their care-givers.

Words, Symbols, and Reality

The main character in this story is a 57-year-old man who lived without feelings. In traditional Freudian terminology, he was obsessive-compulsive. (If you would like to pursue this in detail, we recommend Otto Fenichel [1945] and Lawrence Kolb [1955].)

In this case presentation, it will help to understand certain specific characteristics of persons who are labeled obsessive-compulsive. Such persons do not like to deal with emotional experiences in life. Instead, they attempt to deal with life in a purely rational, logical, intellectual fashion. They are preoccupied with words, symbols, and semantics and avoid the emotional impact of real situations.

The patient lived in a world of words, never going anywhere without a dictionary. He tried to write down all he heard and saw. His pockets were filled with scraps of paper with these odd writings. He was afraid he would forget something if he didn't write it down. He spent most of each day preoccupied with his written messages, which severely restricted his ability to adapt to society. During the last 25 years of his life he was undergoing various kinds of therapy. Despite this treatment, which included electric shock, chemotherapy, and psychoanalysis, he never had a substantial period of relief from his disabling preoccupation.

During his last experience with psychoanalytically-oriented therapy, a curious event took place. While leaving his house one day, he fell down a flight of stairs, broke his glasses and nose, and blackened his eyes. In a way, he had run straight into reality, for during the next three months his preoccupation disappeared and he made considerable headway in his overall problem. But his world of words and symbols returned. This time, though, the therapist had learned his lesson; he wasn't about to return to the usual couch therapy. Instead, he developed a technique of intervention and confrontation in which he psychologically assaulted the man's obsessive-compulsive behavior. After 25 years, progress towards altering the patient's basic approach to dealing with life as real situations instead of symbols had begun.

From the few cases presented so far, it should be clear that changing and altering people is a complex, multidimensional problem. When you approach treatment from only one perspective, the problem may seem insurmountable. Following is another example.

Starvation

The patient was a woman in her mid-thirties. Her primary label was Anorexio Nervosa: she was having trouble taking in and retaining food. In short, she was starving to death. She had gone from 130 pounds to 80, and the staff was afraid she would die. They had tried the usual procedures—talking therapy, chemotherapy, and electric convulsive therapy—without success. In addition to her eating problem, she was extremely agitated. She was considered a big pest by the staff who, concerned about the possibility of her dying, continually gave in to her demanding behavior.

Finally a consultant was brought in. He prescribed a kind of desert island treatment: put the patient in a private room; have her food brought three times a day by an employee who would not respond to her demanding, agitating behavior; minimize her contacts with everyone she ordinarily came in contact with; they were to ignore her eating problem.

Within a short time, the crisis passed. She began to eat. Within a month she was discharged from the hospital. The shift from focusing on the *inner* person to the person's *environment* had had an immediate, dramatic impact on the patient. The treatment isn't new. It was first suggested in the 19th century (Zilboorg [1961]).

New Techniques in Mental Health

Shifting models, as well as gears in our thinking, isn't easy. One of the authors of this book (Fisher [1965]) has gone through a period of reappraisal:

Pychoanalysis, with its techniques of change, has a recent origin. It is

59

not yet one hundred years old. Compared to the traditional techniques of sociopolitical change, which have moved man from despotism to democracy, from slavery to capitalism, and from magical religious thinking to modern-day monotheism, it is a *neonate* [newly born]. These older systems of social organization played an important role when man was struggling with basic problems of existence: slavery, starvation, uncontrollable rage, patricide, and incest. It is unlikely that such problems would have produced psychoanalytical solutions, i.e., turning to insight, understanding, and acceptance. When man faces death or the unknown he more likely turns for answers in such areas as magic and religion.

Psychoanalysis, as a tool of social change, only began to emerge when man began to struggle with problems of freedom and satisfaction, the difficulties of dependence, sexual conflicts, and individuals turning inward to solve their problems. This became an advanced procedure apparently available to the most developed people in the society.

In effect, Fisher was becoming aware that the behavior of man had been modified and altered many times before modern concepts of treatment were ever conceived of in the field of mental health. The theme of changing the inner man is a recent one and is only one of many ways to accomplish the task. In another quotation, there is more evidence of the rethinking process:

We seem to need more public health techniques, treatments that can deal with large numbers of individuals simultaneously, procedures that treat *nonspecifically*. We will not always be able to treat on a continuing basis, so we must be prepared to cope with emergencies. Our goals are more those of symptom remission and reestablishment of basic patterns of personality. It would seem that psychotherapy would be more favorable on an outpatient basis than in . . . large, closed institutions.

The [proposed] program . . . brings into use other systems of social change . . . . Most of the behavioral changes in man as he moved "out of the cave" were brought about by social change—changes in the economy, shifts in political systems, the development of new religions.

It is clear that Fisher had become concerned with the task of treating larger numbers of people under new circumstances. Interestingly, this rethinking developed at a time when he had moved from a clinical to an administrative position. Faced with a broadened assignment from a new perspective, he now thought the traditional clinical model inadequate.

This was a major reconsideration for the author. He had been trained in the traditional, medical-Freudian model in which it was assumed that, in order to change a person, one had to go deep into the *inner man* of that person, determine the cause, or causes, of his problem, and then do something about it. At this point in his thinking, Fisher was considering the possibility of altering the inner man by providing changes in an individual's surroundings. This is the underlying theme of the milieu therapy systems which were developed in the 1950s and 1960s. It would be helpful for you to examine the work of Jones, McGee, and Grant [1952] and John and Elaine Cumming [1962] for a detailed analysis of this model.

Milieu Therapy

Milieu therapy has taken on many patterns in various agencies. The basic concept is that the immediate situation in which one lives plays a major part in determining behavior. It is assumed that environmental alterations change the nature of the patient feedback and thus influence the basic behavioral systems. It is further assumed that milieu therapy can reduce symptom patterns, reestablish the premorbid personality, and possibly bring about major shifts in the makeup of the individual. Accompanying the concept of altering the environment is the belief that mental patients (or any cared-for group—children in institutions, senior citizens in homes for the aged) should play a major role in changing their environment and influencing their destiny.

Patient-Government Movement

This theme of resident participation has led to the development of the patient-government movement in state hospitals. Typically, such patient-government operations are conducted similarly to most large-scale meetings: election of officials, *Robert's Rules of Order*, voting, self-determination within limits. The following from Walter Fisher [1965] describes the operation of a patient-government group at one agency:

Since the winter of 1961 we have been active in initiating, promoting, and carrying through programs of social change in a large state hospital. It is our feeling that these programs have partially helped alter the administrative structure of the hospital; for example, formation of units, and partial

61

blurring of professional roles. Our activities, if labeled, would fall under such headings as milieu therapy, social psychiatry, therapeutic milieu, or administrative psychiatry.

At the time our program was initiated, the institution would probably have best been described as a large, authoritarianly organized, closed, mental hospital. It had a population of almost 6,000 patients; there were several administrators, centrally located, who were forced by the nature of the administrative structure to make most major decisions regarding the lives of the patient population; for example, granting of ground privileges, determining when and how patients would be discharged, to whom discharged, punishment, etc. All direction came from the top; the needs of the patients went for naught.

It was impossible for the staff to react to situations with any immediacy since there was no one available to make quick decisions; for example, a grounds pass took several weeks, discharges, at least several weeks. We could promise the patient nothing, since the person in authority might not follow through on the promise. There was no theoretical system or philosophy to give direction to administrators or therapists. The hospital was dominated by the arbitrariness of those in power. The patient's entire pattern of activities—work, play, sleeping—took place within the confines of the institution.

Into this environment we introduced our milieu therapy program with extreme caution and trepidation. There seemed to be little doubt that any program involved with altering the procedures of the hospital and changing the roles of the staff would create considerable resistance. Persons in charge would be asked to reduce security and accept more blame. Individuals would be forced to lose some authority or to share it with teams. We felt that our program would have to be tailored to the inherent resistance of our facility and the staff. The structuring in the opening phase was along the following lines:

a. We would have two ward meetings held for one hour each. The number and length of the sessions was determined by the staff. There would be one staff meeting each week to train staff and aid the patients in their program.

b. We would have the patients elect their own president and recording secretary. The patient chairman would preside over the joint patient-staff meetings.

c. The entire participating staff would attend all patient meetings. We knew from previous failures with large groups that omitted departments would feel isolated and would assume that others would be gossiping about them.

d. We felt that the staff had to be trained first, so we set up a series of preparatory meetings with the staff before the patient program was to begin. These meetings were used to establish programs and goals for the group. There was much resistance to be overcome; for example, many viewed the patient population as analogous to bad children; there was a tendency to want to punish a patient who insults a member of the staff; and the passive patient was considered the "good" patient. In time, there was a shift toward more patient meetings and less staff meetings.

After eight staff meetings, we made arrangements for our first joint patient-staff meeting. We told them they would elect their own officers; we let them know how many meetings and how long the sessions would last. We had decided that at these large meetings the primary focus would be on ward problems. Personal problems would be discussed in group therapy and individual sessions. As we saw the situation, most of the staff and patients would become bored and impatient if one patient held the floor while talking about his individual problems. At least, in these opening days we wanted to make it as easy as possible for our new team. We felt extremely vulnerable, that it would take little to cause us to lose everything.

This has also become an interesting theoretical problem: whether patients can be treated without entering into specific, or personal, problems. It has been our contention that much of the particulars gathered in case histories and interviews might be useful in intensive-treatment facilities, but in state hospitals such material is rarely used! Treatment systems are generally nonspecific; in this case, the focus was on ward problems rather than personal problems.

We let the patients know that we planned to work within the structure of the hospital. There was to be no struggle between the local staff and the central authority. However, if they had constructive proposals for altering the hospital, we would help them when it was feasible.

The patients held their first election in orderly and efficient fashion. As in most such groups, the opening sessions were marked by griping, complaining, and distrust. They did not like the food, wanted to get out of the hospital, asked why they couldn't see the doctor, and saw no purpose to the meetings. Some felt we were having the meetings mainly to spy on them and felt the note-taking of the staff was proof. The chaplains were accused of being psychologists in disguise. Many of their fears poured out: patients who registered complaints would be transferred off the ward; those who worked would not be allowed to leave the hospital; those without families or places to go to would have to stay in the hospital indefinitely.

We stopped taking notes and oriented them to the basic operations of the hospital. Orientation was a long, continuing process. The staff had to be redundant in orienting procedures. All departments wrote descriptions of their work; a bulletin board with various information was put up; the meetings were used for orientation; a patient committee eventually evolved which helped orient new patients; and the patients wrote up a letter of orientation for all newcomers to the ward.

We were as open and honest in our discussions as possible. It was pointed out that some of their fears were partially true, but when hospital affairs were conducted as originally planned, these things would not have to take place. Many of the problems in the hospital were not directly a function of the formal structure of the hospital; instead, they were more a result of

63

the informal systems. The institution had an infinite number of vacuums. It was difficult to pin down responsibility; most of the staff avoided making decisions, and there was much passing the buck. This was particularly true of the medical staff. There were too few physicians, and most of them were untrained in psychiatry. Many of the traditional responsibilities of the medical staff—for example, giving grounds passes, transferring patients and granting home visits—had become the informal powers of the aides.

In the past we had ignored such vacuums, but we realized that it was exactly these problems that we would have to deal with in administrative psychiatry. So much of the seeming trivia of everyday living had to become the problems of the staff team. Some (including myself) had been off in their dream world doing intensive treatment with a few individuals. In retrospect, it appears easier, but silly, to be preoccupied with specific techniques while Rome burns. The treatment system dragged the staff into the administrative arenas against their own anxieties.

It seemed clear to us that the best way of entering the administrative areas and at the same time providing therapy to the patients was to orient them in substituting constructive proposals for complaints and gripes. We would be helping them meet their needs and possibly altering the social structure of the hospital. (This had been one of our failures with an earlier group. We had not found an adequate procedure for them to convert gripes into constructive problem-solving.)

It was our hope that the patients might take the initiative if they found a procedure for influencing their environment. With an increase in motivation, there might be a greater assumption of responsibility and perhaps active problem-solving. Cumming and Cumming [1962] have suggested that these are valuable therapeutic tools in the large institutions with nonspecific treatment situations. We were substituting modified patient government for the Cummings' work concept.

After the initial phase of griping and expressions of fears, the patients began to make proposals for change. They asked for everything from Coca-Cola machines to changes in hospital rules.

When they had a proposal, they managed it according to parliamentary procedures. If the patients approved it, a proposal was sent to the ward staff. The staff would reject it or return it with the reasons for rejections, or with suggested changes or amendments. This was the first step in giving the patients a hearing as well as a semblance of power.

The patients began to use the proposal system, but they didn't find it easy to give up their long-standing role in the institution. They maintained that they were incompetent and helpless. They held that they could do nothing about their future, demanding that the staff act for them while insisting that they would not get a fair hearing. But the staff remained very much in favor of the patients' initiative.

After four or five weeks, the method began to take. People from outside were invited to the ward: a lawyer to talk on civil rights, a Veterans Service officer to talk on veteran benefits, a representative from Social Security, the chief of the dietary department, and so on.

The changes were not in a continuing, positive direction, however. The discharge of the ward chairman, in addition to the most productive individuals in the group, brought a sharp decline. The group went back to griping, with fewer creative suggestions. But each decline was followed by a new beginning, with the patients formulating new principles as they went along. They wrote their own constitution and developed a new member of the executive branch—a proposal chairman—whose main function it was to present their proposals in the proper form. Innumerable patient and patient-staff committees were formed to carry out the functions that could not be handled by the larger group.

The patients had a long list of activities and accomplishments to their credit, of which I will mention a few:

1. They obtained Coke machines, coffee machines, and public telephones.
2. They changed the bedtime pattern for the hospital.
3. They increased their recreational opportunities tenfold.
4. They developed procedure for securing appointments with the staff.
5. They increased their hospital privileges.

The ward meetings spread throughout the hospital. Instead of one program, there were now 20, and some of them went much furthur than the original ward. There was now a Therapeutic Council, the first real middle-management group in the hospital, which was made up of chiefs of departments, some ward representatives, and assistant departmental chiefs. The Council attempted to deal with problems that were beyond the authority of the local wards; it had encouraged the development of ward programs and had aided in educating the staff. About one-fifth of the patients in the hospital were active in some aspect of the milieu therapy.

The heart of the program were the proposals made by the patients, their attempts to follow through on their proposals, and how these proposals influenced the staff.

There seemed to be little doubt that the proposals would create many new problems and raise much resistance in the hospital. But it is in working through such problems that we hope the patients and staff will grow and integrate.

The patient-government movement has gained major therapeutic or service thrust in the past decade. Patient-government is not limited to state hospitals and residential facilities, however. The disadvantaged, aged, "deviants," addicts, alcoholics, and those seeking help in general have in recent years organized peer-type groups to help them live in the outside community. Examples of this appear in Low [1950], Mowrer [1966], Casriel [1963], and Yublonsky [1965].

Group Therapy

In order to provide a better understanding of community self-help groups, we quote from portions of a stimulating paper by Mowrer (1966) which tells how one small group functioned:

There are indications that the Small Group may largely replace the Established Church. Christianity started as a small group movement with great "therapeutic" power, but it has evolved institutionally in such a way as to become increasingly irrelevant for many modern men and women. Alcoholics Anonymous and residential communties operated by former drug addicts were distrustful of all professionals in the mental health field, for the reason that the latter had so often failed in their efforts to deal with the problem of addiction. And professionals . . . have tended to feel that nothing really very substantial could come from programs which were led by persons who did not have scientific and scholarly training. Happily, the resulting state of mutual distrust and disregard is today disappearing. Self-help groups are, for example, much less rigid than they were formerly in their attitude toward the value of psychotropic drugs in at least selected cases; and many professionals have taken the trouble to acquaint them-selves with the work of mutual-help groups and have often been much impressed.

Integrity Groups (part of the small group movement) function in a very democratic manner and without explicitly designated leaders or therapists. What is said in the following paragraphs applies to the intake procedure employed in what may be called Community Integrity Groups. These are groups which operate on a continuous, ongoing basis, without any formal academic connections, and which are composed of people from the com-munity. Preparation for participation is provided by orientation talks by those who have already had some experience in Community Groups and by written materials. An attempt is always made to provide such groups with "resource persons" or a "core group" who have considerable knowledge and skill in Integrity Group principles and procedures.

Intake Procedure

As a result of personal conversation, a telephone call, or a letter, an individual (on the basis of quite varied sources of information and motiva-tions) indicates that he has decided he would like to be considered for membership in one of our groups. This message is conveyed to the total I.G. community at its next regularly scheduled general meeting (composed of several "groups"); there is brief discussion of the information available concerning this person; if there are no glaring counter-indications, the chairman of the meeting will call for someone to volunteer to chair an ad hoc Intake Committee for the applicant, and then three other members volunteer or are appointed, so that the Committee consists of four persons, usually two men and two women. A convenient time for the Intake Session is decided upon then and there, and the prospect is immediately contacted by phone and the proposed time confirmed or rescheduled. Ordinarily, the Intake is held within the next few days, at the home of one of the Committee members, so that, if the meeting proceeds satisfactorily, the new person can start attending regular group meetings the following week.

These Intake meetings are very unlike a social case-work intake interview. There is no note-taking, and no specific effort is made to obtain a personal "anamnesis" [case history] or "family history," for subsequent "diagnostic" or "dispositional" purposes. "Therapy," in the sense of attempting to help the new person to *change*, *starts at once*; and this is usually in the direction of trying to get him or her to "level" with the Committee, "come clean," "get honest." Different I.G. members have different styles of chairing Intakes, and they may also vary what they do from time to time. For example, a chairman may begin by asking the prospect to describe the nature of the problems or suffering that motivated him to ask for help. In which event, members of the Committee may respond to the newcomer's story by saying, "I can identify with what you are saying," and then speak of mistakes that they have made and the difficulties they have encountered. Or the chairman may start out by himself "modeling," that is, telling his own story. Other members may follow this lead. Eventually the prospect is asked to tell the group something about himself . . . The *sharing* which thus occurs commonly has the effect of releasing, relieving, encouraging, and reassuring the prospect. This puts him at ease and indicates to him that he is with people who have firsthand knowledge of the types of problems that are burdening him. . . . they are not asking him to do anything they are not able and willing to do themselves, and he starts *identifying with them*.

But eventually a point is likely to be reached where one or more of the members of the Committee feel that the prospect is being evasive, inconsistent, or defensive in certain areas; and he or she may be specifically, and very directly, "challenged" on this score. If the prospect divulges the material he has been hiding, that is, he "comes clean," the "heat" subsides and approval and admiration will be generously expressed. And if the prospect seems to feel deeply about his disclosures—fearful, sad, or perhaps deeply relieved—the group may encourage "reaching out." The candidate is asked if he feels warmly toward one or more members of the Committee and would like to go to them, say how he feels about them, and embrace them. Or a member of the group who has been particularly moved by the "work" the new person has done may get up, go over to him or her, and say: "I think you're great!" or "I'm beginning to like you very much!" and embrace the person. There may be a good deal of confrontation and encountering in an Intake, but there is also always a lot of *support*, if and when it is indicated. This is, of course, just another way of saying that candidates are actively

67

pressed toward truth-telling; and when they cooperate, they are powerfully reinforced and rewarded.

If, on the other hand, a person remains supercilious or stubbornly uncooperative during an Intake, if he is intoxicated or medicated beyond a reasonable point, he is likely to be told that the Committee is not satisfied with his performance and is not going to recommend, at least not immediately, his admission to a group; and the process, by which such a decision is reached, goes on right in the presence of the candidate! In other words, he is never asked to withdraw while the Committee deliberates. Rarely, however, is a person categorically rejected. He may be told to make application for another Intake in a stipulated number of months, or sometimes will be asked to consult a psychiatrist, or the Committee may say it isn't sure yet what its action ought to be and will schedule another interview within the next few days.

But if the Committee members feel good about an interview and indicate that they wish to recommend the new person for membership, and if the individual himself indicates that he or she is ready and willing to join and make some "investments" in the group, then the I.G. "contract," that is, the few simple ground rules which govern and structure the activities of our group, is explained.

Ground Rules

1. There is no physical violence or threat of physical violence. Violation of this rule may be just cause for summary expulsion of the offending individual from the group.

2. No one leaves a group session when he is under challenge or upset. Persons freely come and go for any minor reason, but if a person is having a "run" and becomes involved with another individual or the group, he stays on and sees it through before leaving the room.

3. There is no Red-Crossing or rat-packing. When one individual is under challenge, another person does not go to his aid until the nature of the challenge has been made completely clear and the merits of the case reviewed. Also, if a person is spontaneously expressing emotional or moral pain, he is not to be given spurious assistance or reassurance. On the other hand, we are very concerned about justice and never want a group to "gang up" on a member or Intake prospect.

4. There is no restriction as to what language may be used in a group. In fact, persons are sometimes encouraged to use "gut-level" language, both as a means of getting in touch with their own feelings and of communicating their feelings to others. A person doesn't even have to use language; if he wants to he can moan, yell, scream, or make any other type of bizarre sound he chooses.

5. There is no "subgrouping," that is, what is called whispering in grammar schools. If you have something to say, then it is ordinarily said to the group as a whole. Nor is there to be too much one-on-one-ing outside the group. Both procedures drain off energy and content that need to be chan-

neled into the group process. Extended private conversation between members outside the group is to be reported at the next regular group meeting.

6. All conversation and action that transpire in a group are strictly confidential. Members of a group are free to talk about such material outside group meetings with each other or members of other groups in the I.G. Community, but they are not to say anything about another member to a nonmember. (This goes for nonmember husbands and wives and is one of several reasons why we encouraged both spouses to be in the group if at all possible.) Members are, however, free and even encouraged to tell their own story and become more open and honest with the "significant others" in their lives and thus extend and consolidate the greater personal authenticity they gradually develop in groups.

7. And finally, each newcomer is asked to commit himself to the three principles of Honesty, Responsibility, and Involvement—and to be open to challenge in regard to his nonpractice of any of these. He also commits himself to attend six consecutive weekly meetings of the group (allowing for prior obligations), at the end of which time he may leave if he chooses, without so much as explaining why. If, however, after this probationary period, the person continues to attend meetings, he is automatically considered a regular member, with the privileges of occasional absences, if explained and announced in advance.

When our total membership was small, business and policy issues were discussed by the total membership; but now most routine business is taken care of by a Council (consisting of one elected representative from each of the groups comprising the entire I.G. Community and two ex officio members), but the Council is always careful to refer innovations in policy back to the total membership for ratification or rejection. Once a month there is a Saturday evening potluck supper, a purely social event, to which friends and relatives may be invited, but there is no grouping, properly speaking, on these occasions. At our regular weekly meetings, there are, I should say, *never* any visitors. Or instead of the potluck supper, there may be a "talk fest," where matters of general concern are informally discussed.

At the present time, our local I.G. Community has more than fifty members, a circumstance which makes it necessary to have six groups (the members of which are shuffled every three or four months).

Now a word about the *advantage* of having new persons come into the larger group community, or *"tribe"* by way of an Intake Committee.

Advantages of the Intake Procedure

1. The special Intake procedure provides newcomers with a long run, that is, much more time than they could ordinarily have at a regular group meeting. Instead of having a turn of a few minutes or half an hour, the prospect can be the center of attention and concern for two or three hours, or even longer if need be.

69

2. Having been through Intake, a new person comes into the group with considerable knowledge as to how a group operates and some actual, though preliminary, group experience. (A few pamphlets and booklets are used to provide supplementary information, especially "theory.")

3. A point is always made of putting a new person in a group with at least one, perhaps two persons who have been on his Intake Committee. When the individual appears in the larger group, he sees some familiar and friendly faces. This makes him more secure, and often he shows real pleasure at this reunion.

4. The operation of Intake Committees spreads responsibility and experience on the part of group members. Usually an Intake Committee will consist of two experienced and two less experienced members. In fact, a person may be put on an Intake Committee after having "grouped" only a few weeks. In short, it is good training.

A Brief Integrity Group "Case History":

Recently a professional colleague and friend mentioned to me informally one evening when he and his wife happened to be in our home, that he had been seeing a woman with depressive tendencies for some months, felt he was not getting anywhere with her, and said he would like to refer her to our Thursday evening groups. My wife and I agreed that we would be glad to take the matter up with our group at the meeting the following Thursday evening and would ask that an ad hoc Intake Interview Committee be set up for Mrs. Ames (as we shall call her). We suggested to the psychologist making the referral that he get in touch with Mrs. Ames, tell her that he had made the referral, and give her the name and telephone number of the chairman of the Intake Committee, which we would provide shortly after the Thursday evening meeting. If Mrs. Ames felt she would like to have a preliminary conference with three or four of our members about the possibility of attending our regular meetings, she should then call the Intake Chairman and work out a mutually agreeable time for the interview.

I was not on the Intake Committee, but Mrs. Ames—let us now call her Madeline—after she had gone through the Intake and had made a commitment to attend six regular meetings on an exploratory or trial basis, was assigned to the subgroup of which I was then a member. I might say that our entire I.G. Community was then comprised of about 25 persons; and each Thursday evening, after a brief general session, we broke up into three subgroups, which have a revolving chairmanship and which are reconstituted every four months. At her first regular meeting, when Madeline's turn came to speak, she said that in the Intake one of the first questions she was asked was whether she was *hiding* anything from her husband. In response to this question (which she later said neither of her two former therapists had ever asked her), Madeline had said no! But this, she said, was a lie; that she had, in fact, had an extended affair with and then been dropped by

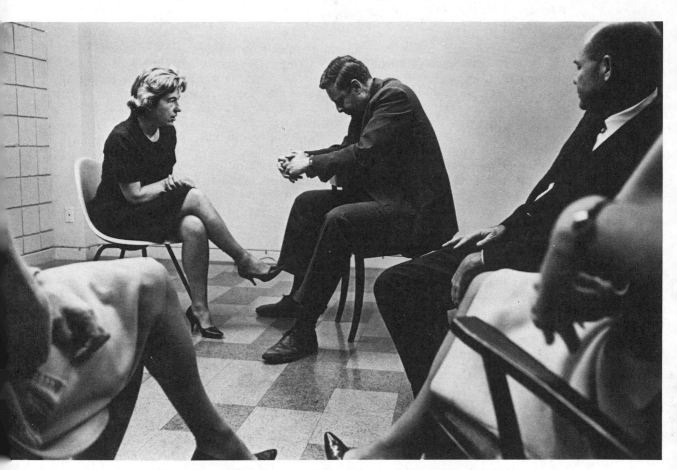

A group therapy session. (Photo by Wayne Miller, courtesy Magnum.)

another young man just before she started dating her present husband, Richard. Richard, who had had a strict religious upbringing, had often talked, during their courtship, of how important it was that both bride and groom come to the altar without prior sexual experience. They themselves, nevertheless had a premarital affair, which was the first for Dick; and Madeline did not admit to any prior experience in this area.

In her first regular group meeting, Madeline said that in the Intake situation someone had asked her: "What do you regard as the worst thing you have ever done in your life?" She said her mind immediately went back to the situation just described. She admitted she had lied to the previous question, and then told a straight story. But she insisted that she didn't want her husband to have an Intake Interview or come into the Group.

However, between the Intake on Sunday and the following Thursday evening meeting, Madeline went through a process which not infrequently occurs. She had found some relief in "coming clean" with the Intake Committee; and she was thrown into a dilemma as to how she should present herself the following Thursday night when assigned to her subgroup, which would consist of seven or eight persons (including one or two members of her Intake Committee). She didn't want to resort to lying again; and she felt she couldn't come in and tell the truth about herself without having first *done* something to improve the situation. So she took her courage in her hands and gave her husband a full and honest account of her premarital history, including the fact that she had married Richard somewhat on the rebound and as a means, so to speak, of making an "honest woman of herself." At times she wasn't sure whether she really loved him or would have married him had it not been for these circumstances; and she certainly had *not* been truly married to him, in the sense of being fully open and honest with him, "of one flesh and one spirit." They had been married 13 years.

When Madeline reported this sequence of events, at her first Thursday evening meeting, she did it in a very straightforward and nondefensive way which made her subgroup respond very warmly to her. And she said that she felt much relieved—and she showed it. At this point she was asked if she felt particularly warmly toward any member of her group and would like to "reach out" and ask for their love (these terms were explained to her). But she declined, on the grounds that she had grown up in a very undemonstrative family and that she just couldn't do this. We explained that this procedure of asking for love often helped emotionally constricted persons get in touch with their feelings—very commonly they wept and experienced a great sense of relief and well-being; but we did not press her to go through with the procedure. However, it was apparent that she had found her interaction with the group very rewarding, as was evidenced by the fact that before the evening was over she had said she would like her husband to have an Intake Interview and then join her group. (When both husband and wife become I.G. members, they have the option, at least in the beginning, of being either in the same or different groups. Madeline wanted Richard to be in her group.)

That night an ad hoc Intake Committee was set up for Richard, who had from the outset indicated his willingness to come into the group. And the following Thursday night he joined our group, which included one of the persons who had been on his Intake Committee. He had apparently not had a very good Intake, in that he was somewhat supercilious and would peremptorily dismiss suggestions or ideas put forward by the members of the Committee. Nevertheless, he told the group that Madeline had been a different woman since she had made her confession to him, that he was more in love with her than ever before, and wished to join the group and would work hard in it.

During the preliminary go-round, which we usually have at the beginning of each subgroup session, Madeline said she had been feeling good, but that Richard was upset and that the two of them ought to have some time later to discuss their situation. After the go-round, the chairman gave Richard the first opportunity to talk. What came out was this. When Madeline had made her confession to him, he reciprocated by telling her of his having once gone to a prostitute, several years ago, when their marriage was at its lowest ebb. This exchange, this mutual confession, between Madeline and Richard had apparently had a wonderfully releasing effect on both of them, and they had arranged to leave their two children at home for a weekend and go for a sort of second honeymoon. Richard was nevertheless mysteriously upset afterwards and went back to see the psychologist who had originally referred Madeline, and had spent most of the hour with him weeping uncontrollably, something that Richard said he had been brought up to believe a *man* didn't do and which was very much out of character for him. Madeline was perplexed by this and showed just a trace of doubt as to whether she should, despite its manifest advantages, have leveled with her husband.

As the work of the group proceeded, this picture became somewhat clarified. Richard was something of a self-righteous prig. It turned out that before he married Madeline, two of his old buddies came to him and told him about her affair with the other man. He pretended he didn't believe them and apparently there were some brief fisticuffs over the incident. He said he really didn't believe this story about Madeline and had put the whole thing out of his mind. She had initiated the self-revealing talk with him after her Intake, by saying: "There is something I want to tell you." And he had said, "Yes, I know what it is." She said, "Then you say what it is." And he replied, "No, it will be better if you tell it."

Thus all along, Richard had something on his wife and was in a sense silently blackmailing her with it—or at least using it to rationalize some of his own less than perfect behavior, including the incident with the prostitute. But Madeline had the character to be severely uncomfortable about the incompleteness and dishonesty in her relationship with Richard; and when, in the context of our Integrity Groups, she had a chance to really clear the whole thing up, she threw Richard badly off balance, and he was beginning to look at himself as the heel he really was, rather than secretly capitalizing on his wife's moral inadequacies. This seemed to put the proper words on Richard's feelings, and he saw the picture *like it was*.

But then events took an unexpected turn. At this point someone went back to the episode of Richard's admitting his encounter with the prostitute and asked him what Madeline had said when he made his disclosure. He said that Madeline had said, "I couldn't care less!" This was obviously a very ungracious response on her part and one which had evidently hurt Richard far more than he had been willing to admit. It took only a little further discussion of this situation for Madeline to ask Richard to forgive her for her poor conduct on this score. Richard and Madeline were soon in each other's arms and seemed genuinely reconciled.

What then came out was that, over the years, Madeline had become pretty domineering in the relationship and often wore the pants. And it also emerged that Richard, although an intelligent and competent man, was excessively dependent upon her, often calling her at work as many as two or three times a day, and trying to arrange to have lunch with her almost every day, at times when it would have been more convenient for Madeline to eat with the women she worked with.

We were now moving down into the area of specific behaviors and laying the groundwork for some commitments to specific behavior changes. When asked how often she would *like* her husband to call her at work, Madeline said *once a day*; and she then added, "And as far as the luncheons with Richard are concerned, I'd like him just to lay off and let me tell him when I'd like to meet him for lunch." Richard accepted these stipulations by his wife as reasonable and wrote them into our Commitment Book.

Then Madeline was asked if she felt she was *missing the boat* in any way, and she said she was sure she wasn't giving enough attention, time, and love to her two children; and she committed herself to spending a minimum of five minutes (and as much more time as possible) each day in the company of her two girls, just *relating* to them.

At this point the question of the preceding week was repeated to Madeline. "Is there anyone in the group toward whom you feel warmly and would have the courage to ask for their love." This time, she looked at one of the older women, got up and walked over to her and stood in front of her and said: "Molly, will you love me?" This woman rose and took the younger woman in her arms and held her closely for a brief time. When Madeline returned to her seat, tears were rolling down her cheeks, and she was encouraged to *let go* and weep freely if she wanted to but she stifled any further emotion. However, she had gone further than she had been able to the preceding week. And at this point, it was suggested that she and her husband again embrace each other. After that, Richard said he too felt very warmly toward Molly and *reached out* to her.

Both Madeline and Richard then took an active part in the discussion of the problems which other persons presented, and when the meeting ended, both of them were radiant and obviously high. But just before the end of the meeting, it came out that Madeline had been feeling so much better the past week that she had gone off the medication she had been taking without conferring with the family physician who had prescribed it on the recommendation of the psychologist with whom Madeline and, intermittently, Richard had been working. We asked Madeline to repeat the name of our groups—*Integrity* Groups—and asked if she thought she had acted with integrity in this matter. She then agreed to go back on the medication and seek to have it terminated or reduced by orderly renegotiation with the psychologist and the physician.

The story of the Ames family is, of course, not at an end, and they will continue to have work to do in the group as long as they are members, which can be for the rest of their lives as far as we are concerned. But they will quickly become *strength* in the group, start serving on intake committees, chairing occasional Thursday evening meetings, and moving into increasingly responsible roles in the total structure of the local I.G. Community and the movement.

Again let me point out that the kind of psychosurgery which occurs in our groups often starts with the disclosure of festering secrets, a process that is often facilitated in the Intake by the chairman *modeling* first and then asking the other members of the committee to briefly disclose themselves in some depth. Soon after the new member moves into his or her subgroup, the guilt thus revealed points to the need for specific behavior changes, and here is where the matter of contract, commitments, and responsibility come in. And then as the members of the group offer their love and support—or express their concern in the form of anger and disgust—the process of involvement begins and grows.

The Sunday following their third Thursday night meeting, Richard and Madeline were at the potluck meal which the group has together once a month, and both of them were in obviously good spirits and said things had been going well.

One year later: Richard and Madeline are still faithful and hard-working I.G. members. Madeline's depression has largely cleared up and Richard has become a *better husband* in many ways. Now their motivation, in addition to continuing to *work on themselves*, is to use their newfound skills to help others.

The Integrity Group model is an excellent example of a peer group community program. It reflects the most recent vectors in the mental health field: community mental health, human services, prevention, and the need for new institutions.

Summary

In this chapter we have provided a sample of problems and solutions human service and mental health workers have come up with. There are as many problems as there are patients, so, if the service worker is to cope with this diversity, he must provide a wide range of services and treatment.

Some problems require treatment, but nearly all require some kind of help. In many instances, people find it easier to ask for psychotherapy, with the implication of being *ill*, than to ask for *help* in the form of love, friends, money, and so on.

If you were assigned to a mental health agency, you might encounter this kind of conversation:

Patient; I need treatment. I am sick and it is impossible for me to go on.

Mental health worker: What's the matter? What are your problems?

Patient: I feel terrible. I cry all the time. It's awful.

Worker: How long have you been feeling this way?

Patient: It's hard to say. Maybe around three months. It's really terrible.

Worker: Do you have any idea what is causing your problem?

Patient: No, I really don't know. It's probably because I'm sick.

Worker: Are these problems interfering with your family life and your job?

Patient: It's an awful situation. I lost my job about four months ago. I can't stand being on welfare. It's a terrible thing.

Such a conversation does not mean the person does not need treatment; more important, he needs *help* securing another position and restoring his basic sense of security and esteem. In this particular situation, he put himself back together and got another job. This is more a first aid than an ultimate solution, but it was unquestionably the high-priority response.

Services should reflect patients' needs and not the wishes and needs of the providers. Experience in the field, meeting clients and surveying their needs, will help the human services worker become more sensitive to patients' needs.

Part II

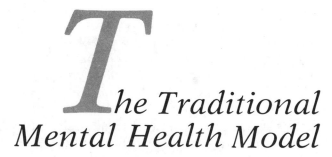

*T*he Traditional
Mental Health Model

Chapter 5 *The History of the Medical-Freudian Model*

S ince early human history, societies have had to deal with the problems of deviance, and mental health systems, like all large social systems, must be viewed in the context of their historical development. Despite its limitations in the contemporary setting, the medical-Freudian model (hereafter called the medical model) has helped society move away from the brutal, sadistic, and inhuman patterns of treatment toward persons designated as deviant.

It appears that from the beginning of human history, all societies have dealt with the problem of deviance. It also appears that the prevailing approaches to deviance during any particular historical period are imbedded in the dominant cultural system of the time. It further seems that reactions to deviance are more a function of the tenor of the times than any other variable.

Preliterate Responses to Deviance

Paleontologists have discovered human remains dating back at least 500,000 years, which include skulls that show signs of a treatment called *trephining*. In man's early history, deviant behavior was believed to have been caused by a spirit, or spirits, inhabiting a person. The preferred treatment was to chip a hole in the deviant's skull, which would allow the spirit to escape and thus eliminate the undesirable behavior. Most did not survive this massive trauma, though there is evidence that a few did live for a significant period of time after the operation.

This treatment and theory are understandable, considering their historical setting. Early man was a primitive, instinctive creature with only a rudimentary understanding of his environment. His lack of knowledge led him to interpret mysterious events as being caused by capricious spirits. He ascribed god-like qualities to rocks, trees, storms, droughts, floods, and so forth.

From the preliterate stone age through man's early recorded history, the theory of deviant behavior was based on primitive religion; it was the province of priests and priestesses. Inhabitation or possession by evil spirits was believed to be the major cause of illness. Treatment ranged from trephining to *exorcism*. Exorcism was an attempt to drive out the evil spirit, originally through prayer, but later by making the deviant person's body an unfit place for any self-respecting spirit or demon. At various times, it consisted of a priest chanting an incantation, administering foul tasting potions and elixirs, and, as a last resort, submitting the afflicted person to torture such as whipping, starvation, or burning with hot coals. These were the major methods until the Golden Age of Greece.

Early Grecian Concepts of Disease

During the 4th and 5th centuries B.C., a Greek physician named Hippocrates lived and worked. He later became known as the father of modern medicine. Hippocrates believed that deviant behavior is a

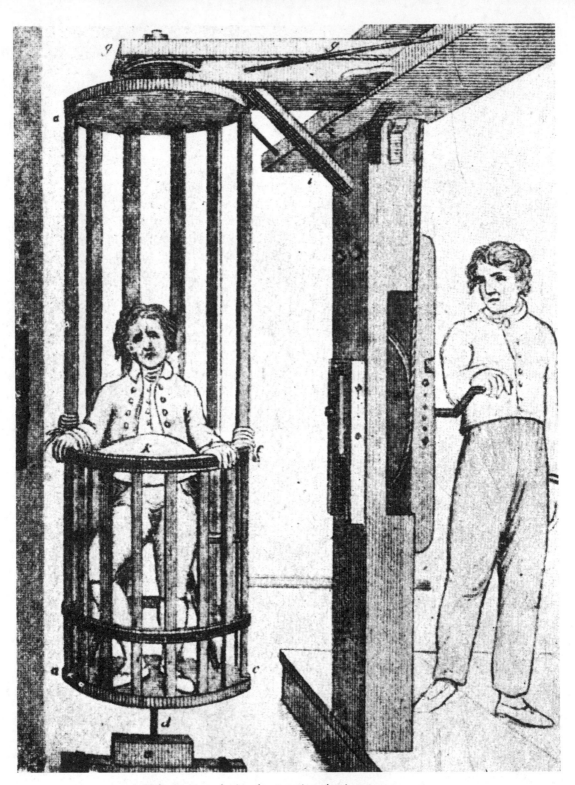

A 19th century device for treating the insane—a "rotator," which was supposed to bring the mentally deranged back to their senses. (Courtesy The Bettmann Archive.)

disease with natural causes rather than possession by demons. He developed a classification system for deviant behavior and prescribed specific types of treatment. Plato, a contemporary of Hippocrates, was among the first to propose that deviant persons not be held responsible for their deviant acts. Plato was among the first to conceptualize the theory of physiological needs, which he called *natural appetites.* The treatment that came about as a result of Hippocrates' and Plato's thinking includes sanatoriums with pleasant grounds, varied activities, special diets, hydrotherapy, and education. Later developments were the distinguishing between chronic deviance, the concept that deviance is an extension of normal traits, the description of phases of mania and depression, and discoveries about the anatomy of the nervous system.

The Golden Age was a period of intellectual ferment and democratic thinking, with oddly enough, a slave-holding substructure. It was a time of relaxed inhibition. The prevailing culture was *nonmystic,* at least to the extent that it supported the search for natural causes of deviance rather than applying a totally spiritualistic approach to the explanation of odd behavior. Many medical advances in the approach to deviance came about during this period. However, these advantages were doomed along with other aspects of Greek and Roman thought when this civilized world was overwhelmed by the barbarian invaders from the East.

The Dark Ages: A Return to Mysticism

In the Dark Ages, man returned to demonology. Greek and Roman advances in medicine were virtually forgotten, and exorcism was again the favorite treatment, though it was now mixed with remnants of Greek theory. Gregory Zilboorg [1941] gives an incantation which was supposedly intended for hysterics and which takes into account Hippocrates' theory of a "wandering uterus" in the development of what later came to be called *conversion reactions:*

. . . I conjure thee, O womb, by our Lord Jesus Christ, who walked over the sea with dry feet, who cured the sick, who expelled demons, who brought the dead back to life, by whose blood we were redeemed, by whose wound we were cured, by whose plight we were healed, by Him, I conjure thee not

81

to harm that maid of God, (name) not to occupy her head, throat, neck, chest, ears, teeth, eyes, nostrils, shoulder blades, arms, hands—but to lie down quietly in the place which God chose for thee, so that this maid of God (name) be restored to health.

According to Hippocrates' theory, paralysis or sensory loss such as blindness were caused in women by the womb becoming unattached and lodging at the afflicted point. The incantation, of which part is given above, was used by medieval priests in an attempt to get the womb to return to its natural place. While Hippocrates believed that the womb moved because of natural causes, medieval priests thought it moved because it was possessed by a demon. As time passed and religion became more rigid and codified, exorcist techniques became harsher. Exorcism changed from benign to malignant: deviants were whipped, burned, chained, and allowed to starve, and ultimately to die.

Those changes were characteristic of feudal Europe. Inhibition and repression were again the main theme of the time. Religious thought was warped by the blinding spiritualism of medieval theology. It became heresy—a crime—to "scientifically" pursue natural causes of physical events.

Witch Hunts

Demonology was combined with witchcraft to bring about a terrifying period in the history of the treatment of behavioral deviance. At the end of the 15th century two monks, Johann Springer and Heinrich Kraemer, published *Malleus Maleficarum* (The Witches' Hammer), which described how to discover, expose, and deal with witches. Largely as a result, thousands of "deviant" individuals were hounded, tortured, drowned, or burned at the stake as witches or warlocks due to the expression of behaviors unacceptable to their culture. A notable example of this technique as applied to an individual who was culturally deviant is the case of Joan of Arc. Her revolutionary ideas were finally stamped out through a process in which the leaders of France convinced the people that she was a witch and had her burned at the stake. This deplorable period lasted almost 300 years, until about 1782, when the last witch was be-

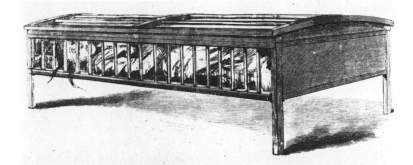

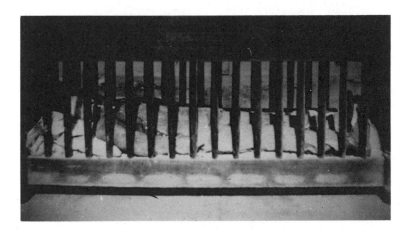

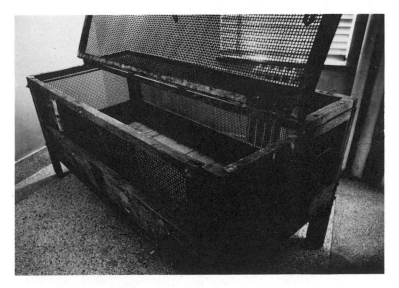

Three views of the ''crib,'' a device used to restrain
overactive patients. At the top is a linecut from 1882, in
the middle is a photograph ca. 1920-30, and at bottom,
photo by Inge Morath, courtesy Magnum.)

headed in Switzerland. This was also the period of the beginning of the Renaissance. Bertrand Russell [1960] succinctly sums up the period:

Social cohesion, during the six and a half centuries from Alexander to Constantine, was secured, not by philosophy and not by ancient loyalties, but by force, first that of armies and then that of Civil Administration. "Christianity" popularized an important opinion, already implicit in the teachings of the stoics, but foreign to the general spirit of antiquity—I mean the opinion that a man's duty to God is more imperative than his duty to the state. What had happened in the great age of Greece happened again in the Renaissance in Italy: traditional moral restraints disappeared, because they were seen to be associated with superstition; the liberation from fetters made individuals energetic and creative, producing a rare fluorescence of genius.

This fluorescence had its impact in a historical period which has been called the First Psychiatric Revolution. In each of the historical examples one sees a correlation between the existing culture and its orientation toward those designated as *deviant*. Early man was brutal, involved in demonology, unconcerned about natural causation, all of which was expressed in his attitude toward deviance. During the Renaissance the seeds were planted for contemporary society and for the current orientation toward deviance.

The First Psychiatric Revolution

Again we quote from the philosopher, Bertrand Russell: "The period of history which is commonly called 'modern' has a mental outlook which differs from that of the medieval in many ways. Of these, two are the most important: the diminishing authority of the church and the increasing authority of science." It is this focus on science and natural causation that allowed a few individuals to begin to consider concepts which became the foundation of the medical model. In the mid- and late 16th century, a European physician, Johann Weyer, daringly espoused beliefs that were antithetical to the prevailing notions of the day:

He was the first physician whose major interest turned toward mental disease and thereby foreshadowed the formation of psychiatry as a medical specialty. He was the first clinical and the first descriptive psychiatrist to leave succeeding generations a heritage which was accepted, developed, and perfected into an observational branch of medicine in a process which culminated in the great descriptive system of psychiatry formulated at the end of the nineteenth century. (Zilboorg [1941])

Slightly over a hundred years after Weyer's work, George Ernst Stahl became the first to propose that certain mental diseases had an organic source, while others had a functional one. Stahl is notable because he made deviant behavior the concern of the psychiatrist. The 18th century was important to this field because it was then that behavioral deviance was finally separated from demonology, and the spirit of scientific questioning was applied to the problem. "The lunatic," said Zilboorg, "became as much an object of human concern as any sick man."

The Beginning of Humane Institutions

Organized *human concern*, of which the behaviorally deviant individual has been the recipient, had its major institutional beginning in the 16th century. One of the earliest institutions for the behaviorally deviant was St. Mary's of Bethlehem (Bedlam), founded in 1547. The *human concern* consisted of mechanical restraint, punishment, poor food, filth, and the opportunity for people to pay a penny to tour the facility much as one tours a zoo today. The over 200 years from the mid-1500s to the late 1700s saw little advance in treatment. In most cases, treatment was so inhumane that it defies belief today. One unusual exception, however, was the Gheel shrine. People believed that a pilgrimage to the town of Gheel in Belgium would provide divine intervention in "madness." Because of this belief the townspeople of Gheel took a relatively humane view toward those afflicted by insanity and began to take them into their homes much as foster parents do today. The Gheel program is still in existence.

The Gheels, however, were extremely rare; harsh incarceration was the rule until well after 1800. In the 1770s a movement began which has become known as the humanitarian reform. Philippe Pinel in France and William Tuke in England were responsible for

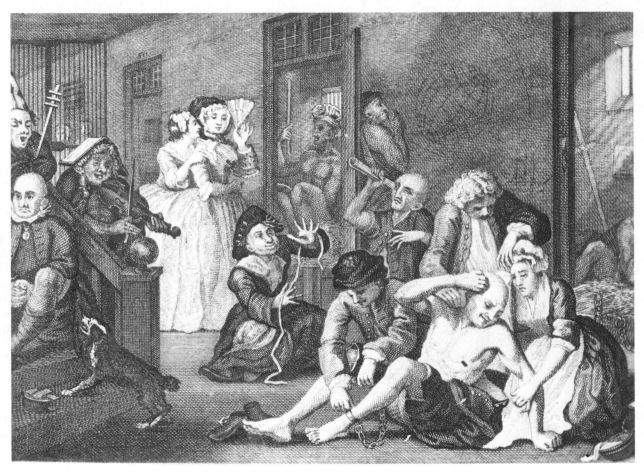

The Madhouse. (Bedlam) by William Hogarth. Bedlam, or St. Mary's of Bethlehem, was founded in 1547 and was one of the first institutions for the behaviorally deviant. (Courtesy The Bettmann Archive.)

starting the movement to remove the chains of mental patients in institutions. The idea that inmates did not have to be chained to walls to keep them from molesting society was revolutionary for that day.

Although there is no question that Pinel's and Tuke's efforts brought about a revolution in the treatment of deviants, the emergence of medical psychiatry during the next 150 years has its own catalog of horrors. Even great figures in psychiatry engaged in what today seems severe and medieval treatment. Benjamin Rush, the "father of American psychiatry," along with Jean Esquirol, a student of Pinel's, was a strong proponent of the *masturbatory theory of insanity*. According to the theory, "excessive" masturbation is debilitating to a degree which can produce insanity. Thomas Szasz [1971a] describes the treatment recommended for women by Dr. Isaac Brown, a London surgeon who was later to become the president of the Medical Society of London, as a clitoridectomy: surgical removal of the clitoris. Masturbatory insanity was established theory until about 1900 and still exists in folklore. Various physicians prescribed castration, clitoridectomy, chastity belts, circumcision, spiked or toothed rings to be worn over the penis to prevent or make painful erections and cauterization or denervation of the genitals. Those notions and concepts, which seem bizarre today, were accepted by nearly all members of the medical profession in the 19th century. This type of treatment has been the fate of deviant persons for centuries.

Dorothea Dix

A major figure in any history of treatment of the behaviorally deviant is Dorothea Dix. While the medical profession was experimenting with a variety of surgical techniques for curing deviancy, Miss Dix, a retired schoolteacher, became concerned about the condition of patients in American mental institutions. In 1848 she reported to Congress that she had seen thousands of persons bound in chains, beaten with ropes and rods, tortured with tricks and "abandoned to the most outrageous violations" (Zilboorg [1941]). Because of Dorothea Dix, public outrage was once again directed toward these conditions, and many reforms were instituted. Numerous hospitals were opened, and their operation was put in the hands of the medical profession instead of stewards or wardens, as had previously been the case.

The American Psychiatric Association

In 1844 a number of physician superintendents banded together to form the Association of Medical Superintendents of American Institutions, which later became the American Psychiatric Association.

While medical practitioners were gathering power in what was to become the field of psychiatry, medical researchers were slowly developing a system of fact and theory which would insure the superiority of the hospital-disease-cure model for the future. Although practitioners such as Benjamin Rush frequently espoused unfounded assumptions, others such as Emil Kraepelin began systematic investigations, concentrating on organic causes of behavioral deviance. Kraepelin was a major proponent of the *organic* theory. He contributed to the descriptive focus of psychiatry by identifying and labeling manic depressive insanity and dementia praecox. Through the efforts of investigators such as Eugene Bleuler, who coined the term *schizophrenia* in 1911, this descriptive labeling approach has resulted in an incredibly detailed system of classification used to identify behavioral deviance. Currently there are over 50 types or classifications of mental disorder listed in the *Diagnostic and Statistical Manual* of the American Psychiatric Association (including that catchall concept of Schizophrenic reaction, chronic undifferentiated type).

The goal of organic theorists is to find an organic cause for all behavioral deviance, in addition to the appropriate medical treatment for it. This approach was given considerable impetus by a number of discoveries made in the 19th and early 20th centuries. A major accomplishment of this period was the incontestable proof that a severe behaviorally deviant condition known as general paresis was caused by destruction of brain tissue as a result of invasion by the syphilitic spirochete. This discovery and the discovery that in some cases mental illness is caused by massive trauma to brain tissue by tumors, deterioration caused by high fever, or certain kinds of severe nutritional deficiencies, strongly motivated research to find the organic cause and cure of all mental illness.

Accomplishments of the First Psychiatric Revolution

The First Psychiatric Revolution peaked about 1900. James Coleman [1972] lists five accomplishments up to 1915 which he considers results of the "first great push in modern psychiatry":

1. The early concepts of demonology had finally been destroyed, and the organic viewpoint of mental illness as based on brain pathology was well established.

2. For general paresis and certain other mental disorders, definite underlying brain pathology had been discovered and appropriate methods of treatment developed.

3. Mental illness had finally been put on an equal footing with physical illness, at least in medical circles; for the first time, the mentally ill were receiving humane treatment based on scientific medical findings.

4. A workable, though not yet completely satisfactory, classification scheme had been set up.

5. A great deal of research was under way in anatomy, physiology, biochemistry, and allied medical sciences in an attempt to ascertain the brain pathology (or other bodily pathology which might be affecting the brain) in other types of mental illness and to clarify the role of organic processes in all behavior.

Whatever else one may think of these accomplishments, they indicate the degree to which the medical profession had become the main force for treating deviance. At a time when most physicians were immersing themselves in the organic viewpoint, a new current of thought was being considered. A few medical mavericks such as Liebeault, Bernheim, Charcot, and Janet had the idea that certain types of mental illness might be caused by psychological rather than organic factors. They were the advance guard of the Second Revolution.

The cultural milieu of this period had an impact on the types of theories to come. In contrast to the Renaissance, which stimulated the First Psychiatric Revolution, the culture of the later period was one that returned to the theme of repression and inhibition. It was

89

the Victorian era and was a period which included the Industrial Revolution and the growth of a large middle class. In most "civilized" countries, the basic problem of survival of the middle class had been met and now the issues of self-satisfaction were coming to the fore.

The Second Psychiatric Revolution

Sigmund Freud must be considered the main conceptualizer of the Second Psychiatric Revolution because of his approach to behavioral deviance. Freud began his career as a neurologist in Vienna and was initially a proponent of the organic viewpoint. He reports in his autobiography that as a lecturer at the University of Vienna he had mistakenly "introduced to my audience a neurotic suffering from a persistant headache as a case of chronic localized meningitis." Freud's point was that he felt he had ignored psychological causality for an organic explanation, due to his organic bias. As a result of his growing dissatisfaction with the organic approach, he went to study with Charcot in France and later returned to Vienna to work with Josef Breuer, a physician who had been using hypnosis on his neurotic patients. Freud's work, mainly with *neurotic* patients, led to a comprehensive psychodynamic theory which began and insured the survival of the movement away from the organic viewpoint. Because it is impossible in the space of one chapter to do justice to any approach or theory, we must be content with a brief sketch of Freudian psychoanalysis.

Freud was a seminal thinker who, through the force of his theories, upgraded the fields of psychiatry, psychology, and social work. We do not mean to imply that these theories began with Freud, only that those he did not create, he justified and rationalized, locking them into the field of mental health.

With his emphasis on the unconscious, Freud [1920] placed the burden of determinism on care-givers. He held that during the first five years, in interaction with parents and people over the issues of socialization, the child develops an irrational, unconscious system, and for the remainder of its life, the child's behavior is largely determined by these unconscious vectors. This was not to deny that with great effort, for brief periods of time, one can change some

90

aspects of the system, but that New Year's-type resolutions quickly fade away under the potent unconscious forces of anxiety, guilt, and depression.

The Freudian position contains a number of patterns. Freud set the stage for an acceptable determinism in the field of mental health. A good deal of the behavior designated as deviant today was encoded in concepts that implied the individual has little or no control over his behavior. While Freud did not ignore or deny the impact of the individual's *life space* (milieu), the determinism was based on the individual's inner dynamics. That is, inner forces are a result of an inborn pattern. But after the environmental forces of the early years, here-and-now happenings have a greatly reduced impact. The unconscious is the greatest source of variance in predicting important human behavior. In establishing the theme of unconscious determinism, mental illness was again placed firmly in the context of a disease. People who act deviantly are unable to stop their deviancy of their own volition which allows the observation that mental illness is little different from a broken leg. Although others saw deviant behavior as perhaps being of organic origin, it was Freud who legitimatized the idea.

There are several interesting implications worth noting at this point. Once the disease concept was accepted, mental health workers became oriented toward curing patients. They wanted to return the patients to an ideal state. In order to cure them, it was necessary to find a cause of the illness, which generally meant a long search into the history of the individual.

The process of diagnosis and treatment was considered to be complicated and lengthy. The therapist had to find access to the unconscious and the past. A diagnostic and therapeutic technique evolved for communicating with the unconscious—free association, interpretation of dreams, interpretation of everyday pathology, projective techniques, and the detailed analysis of case histories. Such techniques are time-consuming; they require considerable expertise and are difficult to evaluate accurately. The focus of the treatment is on the past through a transference relationship with the therapist.

Unless the techniques are handled expertly, the present can be lost and an outpatient relationship with the therapist can evolve which may be lengthy. It is assumed that treatment of the *disease* will be left to the super-elite therapists, primarily the

91

psychoanalysts, and that this treatment is most effective when conducted between two people—patient and therapist. In order to assume this responsibility, the psychoanalyst must be carefully trained, and the training is demanding, lengthy, and expensive.

Patients began to be judged according to their prognosis, a prognosis that was based on their achieving a *normal* behavior pattern by means of analytic techniques. It became fashionable to put the brand *untreatable* on those who did not respond to the analytic method. Most therapeutic systems in this century have adopted such labeling. Those who were not treatable were abandoned.

Summary of Freud's Position

In the Freudian position, behavioral deviance is categorized as a *disease*. Treatment was designed to find the cause of the disease and intervene with an intraorganismic technique. The treaters were to be highly trained, preferably psychoanalysts, and the primary consumers were to be good prognostic risks.

Freud's concepts were controversial when they were introduced early in this century. The ideas of he and his followers, Carl Jung and Alfred Adler, have been embraced by public and professionals alike. Most behaviorally deviant persons, however, have not benefited from this type of treatment. Most deviants were and are being treated in public or private institutions, which have not been able to afford this highly expensive and specialized treatment.

Somatic Treatments

For a long, long time the behaviorally deviant has had few rights. Involuntary hospitalization and involuntary treatment have been the rule. It is estimated that 90 percent of those placed in institutions are there against their will. Meanwhile, the search for quicker cures continued, and a variety of somatic (physical) treatments have been tried on those who are labeled mentally ill.

In the late 1920s *convulsive therapies* were introduced. They consist of a convulsive state induced by drugs such as metrazol and insulin or electrical current applied to the brain, as in electroconvulsive therapy.

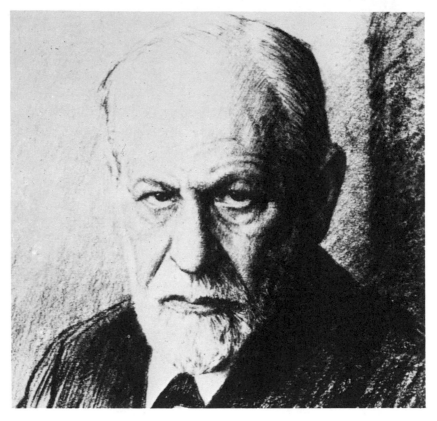

Sigmund Freud during the height of his fame in Vienna.
(Courtesy The Bettmann Archive.)

Two of Freud's most illustrious followers who developed
their own theories of analytic treatment. Left, Carl
Gustav Jung (1875-1962); right, Alfred Adler (1870-1937).
(Courtesy The Bettmann Archive.)

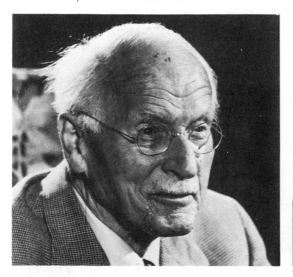

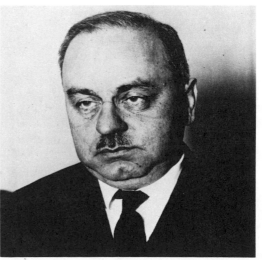

Lobotomy

In 1935 a dramatic new surgical procedure was initiated by Egas Moniz of Lisbon, Portugal. The technique was known as *prefrontal lobotomy* and consisted of surgically cutting the nerve fibers connecting the frontal lobe of the brain with the thalamus. Other, similar, surgical procedures are the lobectomy, the Granthan lobotomy, and the transorbital lobotomy. Ideally these operations reduce anxiety, introjection, inadequacy, and self-consciousness. A number of undesirable side effects have been reported, however, not the least of which is that there is at least a 3 percent mortality rate, and 5 to 10 percent of the patients develop epileptiform convulsive seizures. Other side effects which were reported were distractability, childishness, facetiousness, lack of discipline, and bowel and bladder incontinence. Due to the severity of the side effects, these treatments were used mainly as a last resort. However, over 40,000 such surgical procedures were performed in a 30 year period.

Electroconvulsive Therapy

Another treatment, widely used in the 1940s, 50s, and early 60s, is *electroconvulsive* (electroshock) therapy. It was introduced by Ugo Cerletti in 1938. It also, unfortunately, has some side effects; a short memory loss and mental confusion is common. However, though it has been helpful in clearing depressions, no one is really sure how or why it works, or the effects—permanent or otherwise—it has deep within the brain. Cerletti came to abhor the technique, but it has become a mainstay in public institutions.

Oddly enough, this period of somatic treatments became the period of the infamous snake pits in public institutions. Once again, the question of reform became an issue. Albert Deutsch (Szasz [1971]) describes mental hospital conditions in the 1940s: "In some of the wards there were scenes that rivaled the horrors of the Nazi concentration camps—hundreds of naked mental patients herded into huge, barn-like, filth-infested wards, in all degrees of deterioration, untended and untreated, stripped of every vestige of human decency, many in stages of semistarvation."

Tranquilizers

A history of the medical-Freudian model would not be complete without mention of one of the most recent contributions in the search for cures: the introduction in 1952 of tranquilizing drugs. These drugs were not in general use in public institutions until the mid-1950s, but once in use, they provided a new method of restraint on deviant behavior. Their effectiveness in reducing extreme behavior has had a dramatic effect on the character of institutions. These drugs are effective in controlling about 60 percent of depressions, but there remains a stubborn minority for whom the drugs are mysteriously ineffective. Nevertheless, the staff have become more optimistic, more willing to try new approaches. More patients can be discharged, and hospital populations have begun to decline.

One can see, however, the signs of a Third Revolution coming near on the horizon, and the greater part of this book will deal with its development and structure. The remainder of this section will describe the present system in mental health services (the medical-Freudian model) as the student will encounter it in the field.

Summary

The history of the medical-Freudian model reinforces the belief that responses to deviance are embedded in the cultural milieu of an historical period. Each period has its own assumptions, beliefs, and ideologies, which determine society's view of and response to its deviant members.

Chapter 6 *The Philosophy of the Traditional Mental Health Model*

T he history of the traditional mental health model is filled with beliefs, assumptions, ideologies, and philosophies. The philosophy of the model was discussed briefly in Chapter 5; here it merits more detailed consideration. As a human service worker, you will encounter many mental health professionals in the field who subscribe to the philosophy of the traditional mental health model. While not representing all beliefs, the points dealt with here are, we believe, the important ones in the current traditional mental health model.

Behavior Is Predetermined

It is assumed that behavior is predetermined. Freudians are perhaps the best example of professionals who firmly believe this.

Most professionals in the field, though, have a Freudian training background—psychiatrists, social workers, psychologists, and so on. Advocates of Freud believe that early life events have such an impact on the individual that his later behavior is determined by his reactions to these events, rather than being caused by events occurring at the time of the later behavior. The inner forces in his psyche, which motivate his behavior, are thought to be brought about by his repressed (unconscious) feelings about his relation with *significant others* in his early life. Some examples are given below.

A Young Woman

Sandor Ferenczi [1959] relates the case of a hypochondriacal young woman. The woman was extremely anxious, unable to be alone even for a few minutes. She experienced hypochondriacal bodily sensations and greatly feared death. She believed something was in her throat, that her ears were lengthening, her head splitting, her heart palpitating. She felt that these were signs of her approaching death and had thoughts of suicide. During the analytic sessions she took on the character of her deceased father. She used his name, swearing and giving orders in his style. She even claimed that she had a penis. During later analytic sessions, she acknowledged that she had a six-year-old daughter who was paralyzed from the waist down. The daughter could not walk or control her bowel movements; she required a change of clothes many times a day. She had a strong affection for her child, saying that she loved her "a thousand times" more than her other, healthy, daughter.

It was soon apparent to Ferenczi that the patient was making a great effort to repress her true feelings toward the crippled daughter. In reality, she desired (unconsciously) the death of the unfortunate child. As her husband was away in the military, the pressure on her was even greater. She had to assume the work and roles of both parents, and "therefore took refuge in illness."

The remainder of the treatment progressed along the lines of the typical *psychoanalytic transference* relationship. The woman wanted more than a simple medical response from the therapist and made repeated declarations of love to him. In short, she responded to him on the basis of past relationships with other strong male figures (such as her father). Ferenczi said, "Now, too, I understood the extraordinary fantasy to which she gave expression in one of her pseudo-insane attacks; she again represented herself to be her (insane) father, and declared that she wished to have sexual intercourse with herself."

Ferenczi attributed her gradual improvement to a subtle *resistance* to therapy, an attempt to avoid deeper uncovering of painful material. His analysis of the patient's dreams indicated a paranoid distrust of him as the doctor, that she believed he wanted to prolong treatment merely to continue receiving the fee. At the point the case was finally closed, Ferenczi felt that the woman preferred to continue some of her neurotic "peculiarities."

The Girl Who Couldn't Stop Eating

Another case is from Robert Lindner [1955] in his book, *The Fifty-Minute Hour*. It illustrates the deterministic-nonvolitional assumption system of the traditional model.

The patient was a young, fairly attractive woman who was usually fashionably thin. At times, though, she would go on gluttonous eating sprees which would swell her body to grotesque proportions. Lindner describes one such spree:

The sight was shocking. Everywhere I looked there was a litter of stained papers, torn boxes, empty bottles, open cans, broken crockery, and dirty dishes. On the floor and the tables large puddles gleamed wetly. Bits of food—crumbs, gnawed bones, fish-heads, sodden chunks of unknown stuff —were strewn all about. The place looked as if the contents of a garbage can had been emptied in it, and the stench was sickening. I swallowed hard against a rising wave of nausea and hurried into the room where Laura had disappeared. In the light that came through an archway, I saw a rumpled bed, similarly piled with rubbish. In a corner I made out the crouching figure of Laura. As I turned a light on, Laura covered her face and shrank against the wall. I went over to her, extending my hands. "Come," I said, "stand up." She shook her head violently. I bent down and lifted her to her feet. When she stood up, her fingers still hid her face. As gently as I could, I pulled them away. What I saw, I will never forget. The worst of it was her face. It was like a ceremonial mask on which some inspired maniac had depicted every corruption of the flesh . . . . I closed my eyes momentarily against this apparition of incarnate degradation. When I opened them, I saw the tears welling from holes where her eyes should have been. Hypnotized, I watched them course in thin streams down the bloated cheeks and fall on her nightgown.

98

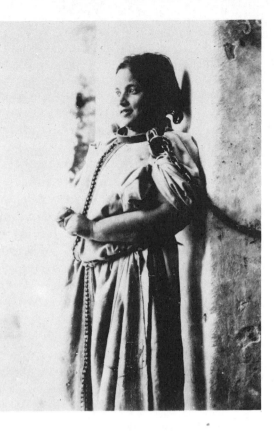

Two examples of the treatment of "mental" patients.
Above an early photograph of a girl in Morocco; below
a present-day scene. (Above courtesy The
Bettmann Archive; below, photo by Bill Stanton,
courtesy Magnum.)

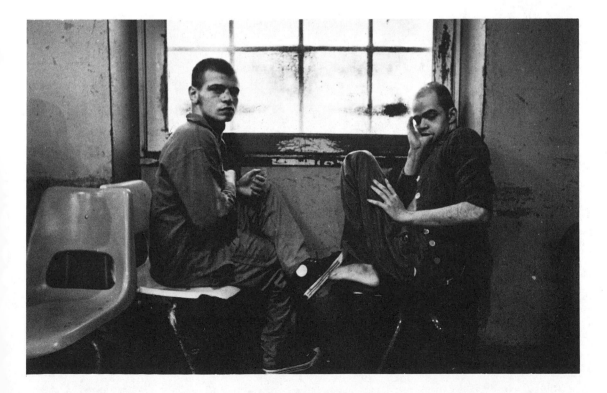

After treating Laura for two or three years, Lindner came to believe that her ravenous eating binges were caused by deep-seated, unconscious inner forces resulting from psychological trauma occuring at an early age. He says: "It was clear that Laura's compelling desire was to have a child, that her feelings of emptiness arose from this desire, and that her convulsions of ravenous appetite were unconsciously designed to produce its illusory satisfaction."

The preceding examples illustrate the deterministic point of view that human behavior is caused by inner forces which are usually unavailable to conscious thought (and usually unmodifiable by conscious desire). An important implication of this position is that an individual is not *really* responsible for his behavior; he lacks volition, or conscious control over his acts. The homosexual prefers men because he identified with an aggressive mother; the obsessive compulsive is overly tidy because he was rigidly toilet-trained; the psychotic is paranoid because he could not develop trust relationships during the first year of life. It seems that for every behavior, at least one *cause* is postulated.

Deviant Behavior Is A Disease

The incorporation of the disease model, as being a response to deviance is considered a major accomplishment by traditionalists. Whether deviance is believed to be a result of deep-seated inner psychological forces, heredity, chemical imbalance in the blood, metabolic disturbance, or vitamin deficiency, the assumption of *disease* and the response to it are evident: the illness is identified, the cause established, and a course of treatment prescribed (see Fig. 6.1).

Figure 6.1 could be expanded indefinitely. For the 60 or more identified *diseases*, there is an equivalent list of *causes* and *treatments*, depending on the theory one subscribes to. Whatever their basic differences, however, the theories have some things in common.

A basic assumption of the disease model is that the mentally ill *sufferer* is unable to help himself. A professional (preferably an M.D.) is required to identify the illness, determine the cause, and administer the treatment, with the object of returning the patient to health.

Figure 6.1

Schematic of the Typical Disease Model Pattern

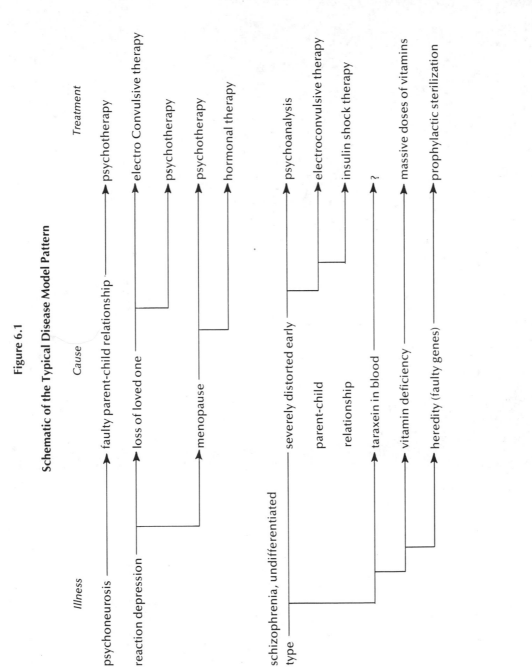

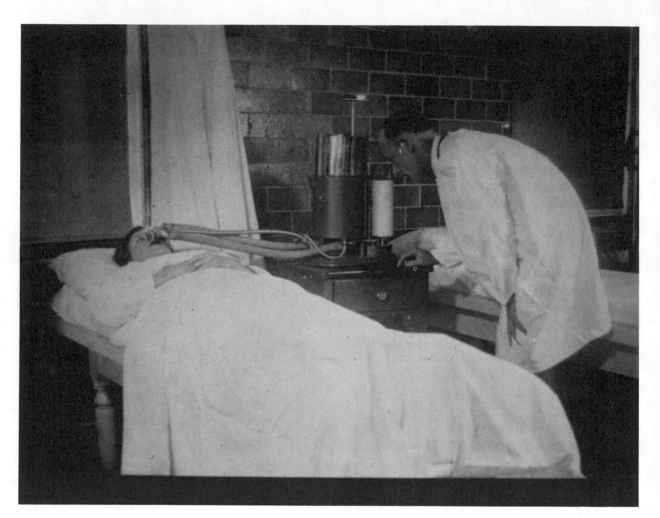

In the 1930s and 40s the search for a physical-disease
basis for deviant behavior often led to treatment such as
this.

Since *cure* by *treatment* is the goal, hospitalization is an accepted aspect of the mental health system. The helplessness of the patient is thought to extend to the point where he may not know what is in his own self-interest. This belief has made possible involuntary hospitalization and treatment. The analogy (from medicine) is that of the contagious disease: an individual with typhoid fever can be legally quarantined and treated even when he does not wish it.

Behavioral Deviants Can Be Separated From The Community

It is accepted practice in the medical model to separate the sick person with a contagious and/or severe disease from his society in order to treat him effectively. The major form of separation (extrusion) consists of admission to a mental hospital, usually some distance from the patient's home. However, extrusion may take on some other forms prior to hospitalization.

Ellen Robertson

Ellen Robertson was a 34-year-old housewife who began having difficulty sleeping and felt fatigued for some months. Rather than showing genuine concern for her problem, her husband told her to see a doctor for some pills for the insomnia. He simply brushed her problem off [extrusion 1]. Her physician prescribed tranquilizers, but they didn't help. During a follow-up visit she began to tell him about her feelings of self-worthlessness and her fears that her husband was cheating on her. The physician referred her to a psychiatrist for help with her depression. During the period of several months that she waited for an appointment, Ellen's depression deepened. She began to neglect the house, and her husband began needling her about her lack of energy. Even after several visits to the psychiatrist, Ellen felt no relief, and her downward spiral continued. She then heard via a "helpful" neighbor that her husband was seeing a young girl from the plant where he worked. An emotional, guilt-ridden scene occurred between Ellen and her husband, and she became even more depressed and immobilized. Her psychiatrist, alarmed at her lack of progress and actual deterioration, suggested private

103

psychiatric hospitalization. The husband agreed. The costs would be covered by insurance. Ellen was admitted to "Mercyland" Sanatorium [extrusion 2]. Her response to separation from friends and family was to become more depressed. The psychiatrist prescribed electroconvulsive therapy, which was unsuccessful. Ninety days elapsed and the insurance benefits ran out, so the psychiatrist recommended transfer to a nearby state hospital 40 miles away [extrusion 3]. Ellen was admitted to the state hospital admitting ward, evaluated as having a good prognosis. A consultant recommended psychotherapy, but no therapists were available, so Ellen was transferred to a somewhat poorer ward since the admitting ward needed her bed for new arrivals [extrusion 4]. She had no visitors but did receive a letter from a relative telling her that her husband was "dating around." She grew more depressed and attempted suicide. At this point the staff transferred her to a "locked" ward [extrusion 5] and her folder was labeled *suicidal*. Ellen was now well on her way to becoming permanently institutionalized. A period of almost a year had passed since her initial hospitalization, and she was more seriously depressed now than when at "Mercyland." During the next several years, Ellen was transferred four times, each time to a more primitive ward with fewer programs. She ended up being diagnosed as a *psychotic* depressive with a poor prognosis [extrusion 6, 7, 8, 9, etc.].

The recent rise in community mental health programs, catchment systems, day hospitals, and such features as family therapy are attempts to reduce the unfortunate extrusion phenomenon. The concept of prognosis, cure, and separation, however, seems a part of the traditional mental health model.

Inner Problems and Adjustment

It is assumed that the current milieu (environment) is an insignificant factor in deviance, that if the individual's inner problems can be worked out, he can adjust to his environment or even transcend it. This assumption is closely linked to the traditional concept that behavior is historically predetermined. Many psychoanalysts, psychiatrists, and other mental health professionals refuse to talk to parents or close acquaintances because they may be part of the patient's inner problem. In one case in the authors' experience, a young man had attempted suicide in his home. His parents rushed him to the hospital and called his psychiatrist to ask him to come to the hospital. The psychiatrist replied that he would come only when the youth himself requested it (which was impossible, since the youth was unconscious at the time). The parents felt both that they had information that would be important in the treatment of their son and that they were being kept in the dark about what was happening to him. Whether this was true or not, the psychiatrist was taking the attitude that the real-life environment of his patient was unimportant in the treatment of his problem. Exclusion of everything except the patient's fantasies, dreams, and memory is common in the traditional treatment approach.

A second consequence of this assumption—many mental health professionals spend considerable time and effort working with their patients to resolve the patients' inner problems in the hope they will reach a "higher" level of functioning. Once the therapist considers this goal has been achieved, therapy is ended and the person returns to his old environment, a process that can result in such situations as these: an adolescent completes psychotherapy and returns to the same family situation in which the problem arose; a child with behavioral difficulties is placed in play therapy, the therapist helps him work through his feelings about his parents, teacher, and school, "cures" him, terminates therapy, and the child returns to the same situation at home and school that existed prior to therapy.

A third example of this assumption which has been operative on a practical level is in the institutional mental health systems of clinics and hospitals. Until recently, their tendency has been to treat patients only when they are within the facility's walls and then only by concentrating on a patient's inner problem(s).

A Black Mother

A black mother with several children and no husband at home takes her one child to a county hospital clinic for medical care. There she waits her turn, which takes six hours. She has no food for the child, receives curt, ill-mannered treatment from a harried staff, is quickly dismissed by an overworked resident physician, and is told

105

to come back for tests the next day. She explodes—yelling, screaming, and throwing chairs around. The police are called and take her into custody. She is anxious about what will happen to her child, hostile toward the police, begins talking about "Whitey's plot against her." The police take her to the local mental health center because she is a hostile "paranoid." At the clinic she is seen by a white, middle-class, male psychologist who helps her calm down and sets up an appointment for the next week. She returns at that time and is given a battery of tests, which indicate that she is of nearly average intelligence, verbal, impulsive, suspicious, fears attacks on the integrity of her self-image. The staff feel that she is a possible candidate for individual psychotherapy with the psychologist who has begun to develop a *relationship* with her.

Therapy begins, one hour a week. The psychologist wants her to talk about her feelings and early life experiences. She wants to talk about her deserting husband, the home she lives in, her child and the possibility that he will get on drugs, the rats in her building, her lack of money, how she has to take the subway across town to the clinic and cannot afford it and ends up walking through dangerous neighborhoods. The psychologist interprets this as resistance to therapy, thinks she is afraid of walking through the "dangerous neighborhoods of her psyche." The sessions continue. The woman's husband shows up at home and moves back in. Welfare workers discover this and discontinue her aid-to-dependent-children (ADC) funds. She is upset and calls the therapist who tells her to talk about it at their next session. He doesn't want the feelings "leaked" over the phone; besides, she might come to depend on the phone calls. The woman is annoyed by the psychologist's response but walks to the clinic for the next session.

During the session, she is keenly interested in getting back on ADC from the welfare department and wants the psychologist to help her. He asks her about her *feelings* about her husband coming home and suggests that she may lose her welfare support if he does it again. She wants action. The psychologist tells her that that is not his role. She accuses him of tricking her, of being against her just like the others. In a rage she runs from the office, slamming the door with such force that the glass shatters. She never returns for her sessions but does, of course, return to the ghetto. The psychologist closes the case with a summary describing her as extremely impulse-ridden, resistant to therapy, lacking in insight, suspicious of those who desire to help her, and paranoidal, with a poor prognosis. Even had he cured her, the end result would most likely have been the same: she would have returned to the same situation she came from —public aid, dependent children, county hospital clinics, rat-infested rooms, and so forth.

This example can be extended to illustrate the effect of the basic assumption in the hospital situation. Following her withdrawal from the clinic sessions, angry, hostile, and suspicious, she makes repeated attempts to have her welfare money reinstated. Public aid workers respond to her angry threats and "paranoidal" allegations by having her taken by the police to the state mental hospital. Following an admission examination, which *confirms* her *paranoidal ideations* and high level of anger and hostility, she is persuaded to voluntarily sign into the institution and is transferred to a ward. The social worker of the ward subsequently obtains her clinic history folder; as a result of the psychologist's negative remarks in her clinic history, the social worker feels that the patient would not benefit from *talking therapies*. The patient is placed on tranquilizing drugs, and her symptoms are gone in a short time (several months). During the course of her hospitalization, a complete social history is done, which outlines her occupation (none), family relationships (few), and social patterns (lacking). She is not considered a good *therapy* case, so little more than chemotherapy is tried. She is released and again placed on public aid. Following her release, she gets her son (who stayed with a cousin) and returns to the ghetto. Her environment is now the same as it was prior to hospitalization—the same frustrations, same resources (none), same problem. There is only one change: she is now considered mentally ill, with a poor prognosis.

This example is typical of the mental health field in recent years. A few attempts have been made to deal with the environment but they are in the minority—generally family therapy, crisis intervention, sheltered-care facilities. The main focus remains, however, on the inner individual rather than the factors in his environment that precipitate, cause, or aggravate his deviant behavior.

Elite Training

It is assumed that treatment is so complex that only highly trained, specially qualified, persons are equipped to utilize it. It has been traditionally assumed that in order to be a physician, one must undergo long years of training—an appropriate assumption *in the medical context.* But the same assumption has been applied to *credentials* in the traditional mental health field. The longer the period of training and the more complex its contents, the greater the prestige of the worker. This system is reflected in the salary levels of employees in the field. If one were to rank the professions on the basis of their worth, it would probably look like this:

1. psychoanalyst
2. psychiatrist
3. physician
4. psychologist (Ph.D.)
5. social worker (N.A.S.W.)
6. psychologist (M.A.)
7. psychiatric nurse (M.P.N.)
8. activity therapist (M.A.)
9. occupational therapist (M.A.)
10. all other master's-level personnel
11. bachelor's-level personnel
12. psychiatric attendants

This attitude is so pervasive that it has been incorporated into our language: a psychoanalyst without a medical degree is a *lay* analyst; a professional without a medical degree is an *ancillary* staff member; a staff person without at least a master's degree is a *paraprofessional.* The idea that by becoming generalists we become less than professional is perhaps the crux of the matter. We suggest that one does not need a *professional* degree to be professional. While it is true that advanced degrees are required in such activities as psychoanalysis and intensive psychotherapy, there are a myriad therapeutic or helping endeavors that can be successfully accomplished by the *nonprofessional,* perhaps far more than realized.

Medical Authority Is The Ultimate Authority

The assumption that medical authority is ultimate is a corollary to the preceding assumption. The use of the medical-disease model has resulted in the adoption of this idea. Most governments (local, state, and federal) have legislation on the books which requires administrators of departments of mental health, superintendents of hospitals, and directors of clinics to be medical doctors. The requirement for occupancy of the position has become one of *credentials* rather than *competence*.

Medical authority is considered final in diagnosis, treatment, privileges, discharges, and, in some cases criminal responsibility. It is accepted that the medical doctor has expertise that other members of the staff do not. The lack of physicians then leads to situations which compound the problem of leadership. The following excerpt from *Critical Mass #1* (Fisher, Mehr, and Truckenbrod [1971]) illustrates a situation that has developed as a result of power residing in the hands of a select few:

Afraid of criticism, they left decision-making in the hands of the "super" experts. In our agency, three men, all in administrative positions, infrequent visitors to the wards, made most [of the] formal decisions regarding the operation of the hospital and the fate of the patients. Even with these men having the best credentials, the superintendent felt he had to review all of their decisions. Assuming that these men had the wisdom to make appropriate judgments, they were overwhelmed by the size of the task—the vicious circle. If any of the administrators became ill or went on vacation, the already staggering system would approach collapse. Important decisions would be delayed or never made and the patients who might have been quickly moved through the system were held and institutionalized.

The belief that medical authority is *the* authority is so pervasive in our culture that even the judicial process has in many instances bowed out of the decision-making process and deferred responsibility to the psychiatric profession. Commitment to a mental institution on the grounds of being incompetent to stand trial for a crime is relatively common today. The decision of incompetence is made by a psychiatrist; the patient remains *incompetent* until another

109

psychiatrist feels he is sufficiently recovered to return to court. In his book, *Law, Liberty, and Psychiatry*, Thomas Szasz [1963], examines this situation in depth.

Traditional Concepts, Assumptions, and Misconceptions

The following list, while not comprehensive, is illustrative of the current types of concepts, assumptions, and misconceptions of the medical model:

Patients who do not respond to therapy are probably untreatable. This leads to a labeling process resulting in categorizing persons as having poor prognoses. It places the responsibility on the patient, fixes blame, and exonerates the therapist. It has far-reaching effects, insuring that in subsequent *therapeutic* situations, the patient will begin with at least one strike against him.

Mental illness may be so severe that patients are not responsible for their behavior. In many cases, this belief allows strong, positive reinforcement of deviant behavior; criminality is excused, acting out is accepted. In addition, it allows society to lock up persons it thinks are incompetent and to remove their control over personal possessions such as money and home.

Patients must frequently be GIVEN treatment even though they do not want to be treated. This is related to the irresponsibility issue, the belief that patients frequently do not know what is in their own best interests. No matter how they protest, if the doctor believes that they are sick, they are forced to accept treatment, whether they like it or not.

Insight is necessary for growth. Most therapeutic systems are based on the belief that insight is a prerequisite for growth, satisfaction, or normalcy. Many times this is not so. The policeman, soldier, butcher, factory worker, mental retardate, etc., may, in fact, experience a decrease in his ability to function if he experiences true insight.

Schizophrenics have little sexual desire; schizophrenics have an overabundance of sexual desire. Both assumptions are common. Programs and administrative decisions have been made based on both assumptions in different situations. In some institutions the sexes are continually segregated for the second reason; in other situations sexual activity is seen as a healthy step forward, based on the first assumption.

Epilepticism and psychosis cannot occur in the same personality. Epileptics cannot become schizophrenics, and vice versa. We do not know where this myth started, but diagnoses have been made on the basis of it. Schizophrenics who have had epileptic seizures have sometimes been routinely diagnosed as malingerers.

Schizophrenics have developed their behavior patterns because of being reared by schizophrenic mothers. According to this assumption, mothers with a particular type of personality are unable to form a healthy relationship with their children which results in the children developing schizophrenia. The assumption fails to take into account the large number of mothers who have this personality type whose children *do not* exhibit behavioral deviance. Occasionally, the assumption is turned around: mothers of schizophrenics must have this personality type.

Summary

In this chapter we have shown how the traditional mental health model with its emphasis on predetermined behavior and the concept of prognosis, cure, and separation from the community, has dominated the mental health field since Freud. In this model, the environment is considered an insignificant factor in deviance and patients have been traditionally separated from society for treatment with neither the family nor the milieu considered part of the therapy. The medical authority is in command in this context with highly trained and certified personnel forming the rest of the staff. From this background, various assumptions and misconceptions have arisen over the years which further confuse and prevent proper treatment.

Chapter 7 *The Organization of the Traditional Mental Health Model*

We now turn to an examination of the organizational system that prevails in most mental health agencies today. In many respects, the organizational system which exists in an agency has an important facilitative or restrictive effect on the character and effectiveness of the programs implemented. In the traditional mental health model, the use of the medical-disease-cure model for treating behavioral deviance has led to a situation in which the prevailing organizational system bears a strong resemblance to the general medical model. This system is usually called the *authoritarian* model and is the system the human service worker is most likely to encounter in the field.

The Authoritarian-Pyramidic-Departmental Model

For a long time, the dominant organizational model in mental health has been the authoritarian-pyramidic-departmental (A-P-D) model. In it, a few individuals hold and maintain power and authority because of their supposed expertise, while at the same time being the furthest removed from actual contact with the patients. Figure 7.1 is an organizational chart showing this type of organization at an inpatient psychiatric institution. Both public and private inpatient institutions are usually organized along the lines indicated in the chart. There is a nearly direct inverse relationship between a worker's position in the organizational table and his position relative to the patients. Directors seldom see patients; department heads see patients only in special situations; disciplinary staff see patients for short periods of time each day; and nursing-ward staff such as aides and attendants see patients throughout the workday.

The only staff with responsibility for total treatment programs are the nursing staff, which are frequently the only staff assigned directly to a specific ward area. Other staff are assigned to their departmental supervisors rather than to patient areas, which produces a situation in which the staff who appear in a ward work for a short period and report to as many different supervisors as there are types of personnel in the ward—social work, psychology, activities, physicians, nurses, aides, and so on. Since the nursing staff (nurses and attendants) have the major responsibility for the patients' welfare, we should examine the organization of the nursing service. (Figure 7.2 is an extension of Figure 7.1 and presents the typical organization of the nursing service.)

The A-P-D model is limited by its structure. Decision-making is remote from the patients, decisions that affect the patients' life style—whether they will be allowed home visits, grounds and off-grounds passes, or whether they are sufficiently recovered to be discharged. Since the authority for making these decisions is far removed from the patients affected, there is a considerable potential for error.

113

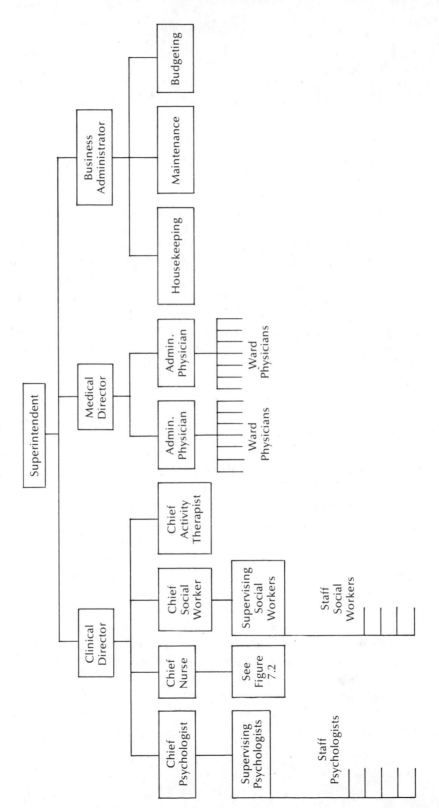

Figure 7.1

**A Typical Organizational Structure of an
Inpatient Psychiatric Institution**

Figure 7.2

**Organization of the Nursing Services
in a Typical Inpatient Psychiatric Institution,
with the Focus on the Day Shift**

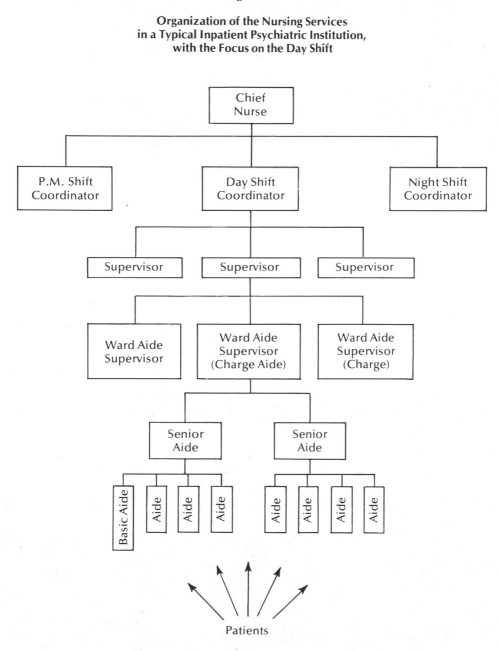

Patients

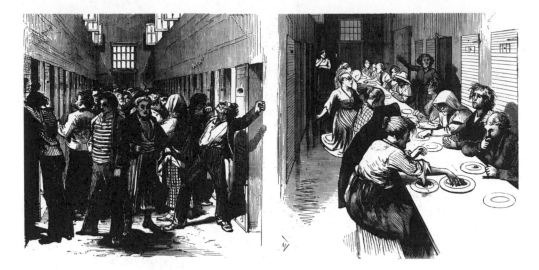

Scenes from the insane asylum of old Blockley Hospital
in Philadelphia. Institutions such as Blockley were the
forerunners of today's authoritarian-pyramidic-
departmental model. (Courtesy The Bettmann Archive.)

Engraving depicting a crowded ward of the
Lunatic Asylum at Blackewell's Island in New York in
1868. Note the lone ward attendant. (Courtesy The
Bettmann Archive.)

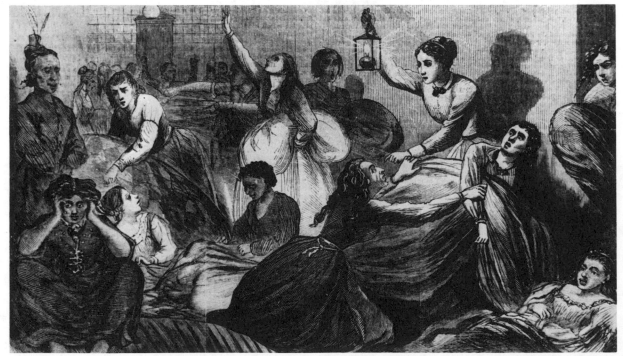

When a patient wants a privilege, he must request it from a staff person on his ward. In most cases, psychology, social work, and activities staff do not have easy access to the decision-making process, so if the patient makes his request to them, he is referred *back* to the nursing service. The patient's main contact is with the ward aides, to whom his requests are usually made. The ward aide sends the request to the senior aide; the senior aide passes it on to the ward aide supervisor or charge aide who notes the request and brings it to the attention of the physician. The physician forwards it, if he so chooses, to the medical director and the clinical director. Then the medical director, clinical director, and superintendent meet to evaluate the case and make their decision, basing that decision on information that has been gradually altered by five levels of referral. At any point in its progress, the request can be rejected and turned back, but it can be given approval only at the *top* administrative level of the institution. When the process works well, it takes three to four weeks; when it doesn't, months pass.

When any of the three top men at one hospital organized around this model—the superintendent, medical director, or clinical director—becomes ill or takes a vacation, the decision-making process stops. In some cases, three months have passed before a decision was made.

Because of this system, privileges have often been withheld from patients who could have handled them, and patients who could have been discharged have languished in wards for months. The system, in short, is conservative; it abhors taking risks. It tries to avoid errors simply by making as few decisions as possible. Sins of *omission* are not punished; sins of *commission* are. If a patient does not receive privileges he is well able to handle, no one is concerned. However, if privileges *are* given to patients who later encounter difficulty in handling them, the staff is reprimanded. A patient who could be discharged but is not causes no problem in the system. A patient who is discharged and who then behaves poorly causes considerable pain to the system, which, in turn, causes those using the authoritarian model to err on the side of safety and security.

There are other limitations of this model resulting from the centralization of services in both the budgetary and program areas. In the traditional authoritarian system, budgetary services are separate from clinical systems. Personnel needs, equipment needs,

117

remodeling needs, construction needs, and so on are reviewed by a business administrator who makes the final decisions as to how much and in what way money will be spent. But here a major problem often develops: the administrator is often unfamiliar with clinical services and thus makes his decisions on purely fiscal grounds. Clinical staff, including the superintendent, are naive about what can and cannot be done with the money available; frequently they are uninformed about *how much* is available.

The centralized budgetary process has led to a variety of problems in fiscal management in institutions. In a large midwestern state hospital a few years ago, the director (of a centralized business administration service) felt that it was his job to limit spending and return unspent funds to the state. As a result, only a small percentage of the available maintenance and remodeling money was spent. Monetary requests were buried in red tape and eventually not approved. The physical plant of the hospital slowly deteriorated; wards became grimy, outmoded, almost uninhabitable. The business administrator, of course, achieved his goal: he returned thousands of dollars to the state. Economy came first, clinical and patient priorities second.

Centralized patient services are linked with the departmentalization of disciplines, to list another limitation of the A-P-D model. Since the institution is organized on departmental lines—for example, social work, psychology, activity therapy, occupational therapy—services tend to be delivered to patients along the same lines. The delivery is directed by a central authority. Rather than have comprehensive treatment programs developed in the wards, with program and decision-making responsibility given to the staff, the various members of the staff work for their department supervisors, moving to wards only when they are to perform their specialized functions. The reverse occurs when a patient leaves the ward for a specified period of time to go to a central treatment point such as an activity and recreation center or a rehabilitation workshop. The responsibilities of the patient are effectively fragmented: the psychologist is in charge of his inner self; the social worker is in charge of his family relationships; the hospital is in charge of communication with his relatives; the activity therapist is in charge of his avocational interest; the rehabilitation counselor is in charge of his work activity. The departmental staff share information with

118

others in their own department, but due to the nature of the system, information between departments is rarely shared.

The Class and Caste System

In the traditional mental health model there is a class and caste system which is most evident in the A-P-D model. There appears to be a direct correlation between one's level in the hierarchy and the degree of relatedness with patients, between level and discipline, and between level and prestige. Although in actual practice, there is some overlap of function, level, and discipline, the A-P-D model follows the structure shown in Figure 7.3. The categories near the top have the greatest prestige; those at or near the bottom have the lowest. In this system, the patient, of course, has the least prestige; he tends to be treated as an object to be manipulated.

Staff functions in this class and caste system are defined horizontally and rigidly proscribed: the ward aide cannot do activities with the patients; the activity therapist cannot do a social history; the social worker cannot do psychological testing; the psychologist cannot make discharge decisions. The system virtually guarantees that no one will want to engage in functions of the next *lower* level; it would be demeaning and cause loss of status.

This system results in further fragmenting of communication systems, as well as a system rife with envy, jealousy, and antagonisms. The major schism is between the professionals and the nonprofessionals. The two camps regard each other with suspicion and animosity. Usually the professional group is defined as those with advanced education, while the nonprofessional group are those with a high school diploma or less. The system generally does not employ many who have been to college. The two camps view each other with suspicion and the atmosphere is generally not conducive to cooperation.

Systems in Transition

In the discussion thus far, we have dealt mainly with what has been the typical organization model of public and private mental

Figure 7.3

The Hierarchy of Disciplinary Class and Caste

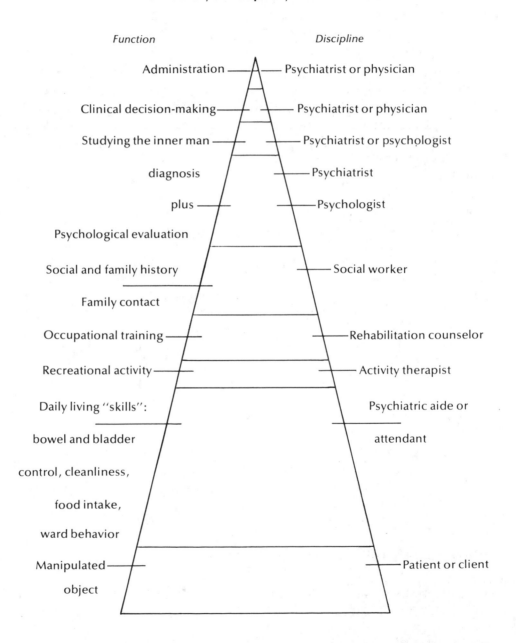

Function   *Discipline*

Administration —— Psychiatrist or physician

Clinical decision-making—— Psychiatrist or physician

Studying the inner man —— Psychiatrist or psychologist

diagnosis —— Psychiatrist

plus —— Psychologist

Psychological evaluation

Social and family history —— Social worker

Family contact

Occupational training —— Rehabilitation counselor

Recreational activity —— Activity therapist

Daily living "skills":   Psychiatric aide or

bowel and bladder   attendant

control, cleanliness,

food intake,

ward behavior

Manipulated —— Patient or client

object

health institutions. For many decades the organizational systems have been static, but in recent years there have been some organizational changes, although most have not reached the point where they can be considered representative of a *human services* system. Louis Rowitz and Leo Levy [1971] discuss a number of the transitional phases of changing organizational systems in institutions in mental health. While working for the Illinois Department of Mental Health Division of Planning and Evaluation Services, they described five stages of reorganization in institutions: (1) the centralized hospital model (equivalent to the basic A-P-D system); (2) the centralized transitional model; (3) the subhospital model; (4) the decentralized transitional model; and (5) the decentralized hospital model. The most prominent characteristics of these stages are given in Table 7.1. They will be encountered by human service workers in various settings since hospitals and clinics are in quite different points in the continuum of reorganization.

Our focus here will be on the fifth stage in Rowitz' and Levy's schema, a stage which has become more and more common in current mental health systems. It is considered by many to be the ultimate in organizational design, but we feel that it still includes a number of the pitfalls of the A-P-D model.

Stage five is the decentralized hospital model, in which the institution is broken down into programs, usually on a geographic (county) basis, with a small number of specialized treatment programs such as geriatrics, medical-surgical, alcoholism, and children's and adolescents' programs. Figure 7.4, also from Rowitz' and Levy's article, is an organizational chart of this type of setting. In it, power and authority lie in the hands of the program director, or *unit chief*. He has administrative responsibility. Each of his wards is under the control of a multidisciplinary team which reports to him through a team leader. Department heads have little power, having no line authority. If department heads do stay on, they do so as anachronisms, with only staff roles in recruitment, training, and consultation. In one hospital, the department heads disappeared after this type of organization was introduced.

One effect of such a reorganization is to "flatten" the authority pyramid. Decision-making responsibility is placed at a lower level in the system. Decisions concerning such issues as patient privileges and discharges usually occur at the team level. Those making the

121

Table 7.1
General Characteristics of Five Conceptual State Mental Hospital Models on the Centralization-Decentralization Continuum*
(from Rowitz and Levy, 1971)

Hospital model	Organizational Structure	Formal communication pattern network	Service chiefs' authority	Treatment orientation	Admission procedures	Discharge procedures	Readmission procedures
Centralized hospital	Centralized administrative services or departments	Vertical-line authority communication possible among service	Line-direct supervisory control over all members of discipline	Custodial	Centralized	Centralized	Centralized
Transitional, centralized hospital	Centralized administration with specialized programs	Generally vertical with horizontal communication possible in programs and services	Same as above; some conflict between department heads and program chiefs	Custodial, with a few therapeutic treatment programs	Centralized with staff referrals to special programs	Centralized with direct discharge from program wards	Centralized with possible reassignment to special program ward if patient was on it before
Subhospital	Large "program"-oriented hospital subdivisions (little coordination among subdivisions)	Vertical and horizontal within subdivisions; blocks between subdivisions and also between subdivisions and administrative staff	Line authority, however, difficulty in supervision of staff once assigned to the subhospital†	Treatment orientation may be custodial or therapeutic	Either centralized or decentralized	Direct discharge from subdivision	May be centralized or decentralized
Transitional, decentralized hospital	Initial development of units from subhospitals	Horizontal with communication blocks between units and also between units and administrative staff	Line authority role breaks down, for service chiefs have difficulty in finding new role	Therapeutic orientation, with transition implementation difficulties	Decentralized to unit admissions service	Direct discharge unit	Readmission to same unit as on previous admission
Decentralized hospital	Decentralized administration geographic catchment units with coordinating councils and units	Horizontal within units, vertical between coordinating councils and units	Staff role in recruitment, training, and professional consultation	Therapeutic	Decentralized to unit admissions service	Direct discharge unit	Readmission to same unit as on previous admission

122

*In this table, we are describing a theoretical approach to hospital decentralization for large mental institutions. A small hospital may find it organizationally expedient to remain centralized but to have a therapeutic treatment orientation.

†Subhospital may establish service chief positions for the subhospital.

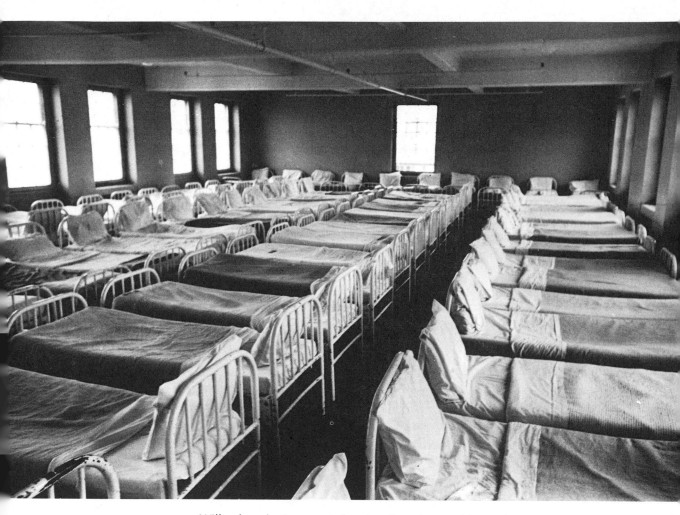

Willowbrook. A present-day dormitory in a residence for
the mentally retarded. Photo by Bill Stanton, courtesy
Magnum.)

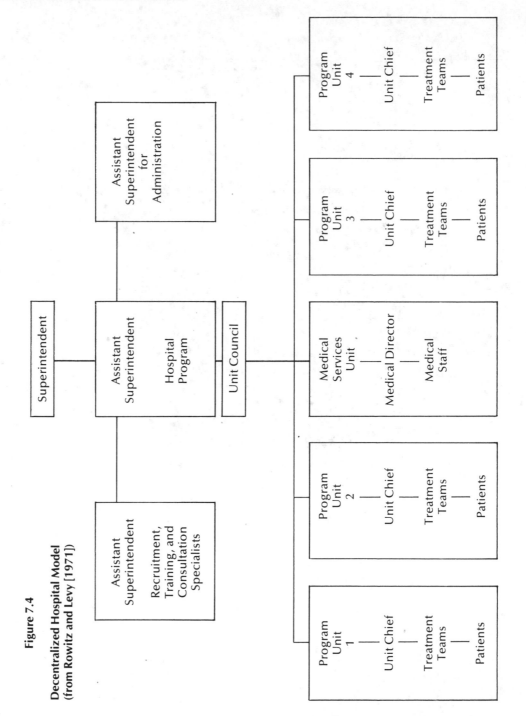

Figure 7.4

Decentralized Hospital Model
(from Rowitz and Levy [1971])

decisions work with the patients and know them. They seem more willing to take risks than would a distant triumvirate, as was the case in the A-P-D model. In one institution, where once all decisions were made by the top three administrators, currently more than 50 teams make the decisions. The time lag between request and action has been reduced dramatically.

Besides clinical decision-making and programming, many institutions have initiated program budgeting, in which program directors or unit chiefs take a major part in the preparation of budgets. Within broad guidelines, the program director has virtual carte blanche in deciding how to use his budget and how best to meet the fiscal needs of his patients. This type of system allows innovation, although it does not guarantee it.

At least one major difficulty remains in this type of system: emphasis is still on disciplinary expertise. Under the basic team concept, each specialist contributes his knowledge to the team, and the whole team brings it together. In actuality, the patient's relationships remain fragmented among the members of the team. The class and caste system remains implicit in the system.

The Rowitz and Levy schema is based on the mental health scene as it was in 1968. There have, of course, been dramatic changes in organizational style since then, at least in some settings. The changes subsequent to 1968 begin to more closely approach the kinds of organizational systems appropriate to a human services network and will be dealt with in section IV of the book.

Summary

The organizational system which exists in an agency can facilitate or hinder the programs implemented at the agency. A five-step system was presented, which characterizes inpatient facilities on the basis of a centralization-decentralization continuum.

Centralized agencies tend to be departmentally-oriented and authoritarian in nature while decentralized facilities tend to be the opposite.

A typical problem in the authoritarian system has been the distance between the decision-makers and the patients most directly affected by these decisions.

Chapter 8 *Traditional Mental Health Delivery Systems*

Traditional mental health delivery systems consist of an organizational network through which services are provided; professionals deliver the services, and patients receive the services. Most mental health delivery systems today have grown out of the private, entrepreneurial medical model. In this type of system, a person with physical discomfort, pain, or sickness purchases diagnostic and treatment services from a licensed medical practitioner. In other words, he enters into a patient-doctor relationship.

It has been assumed that the same system is appropriate for mental health services. In private-practice situations, people who feel *psychic* pain go to licensed psychotherapeutic practitioners such as psychiatrists, psychologists, psychoanalysts, or social workers and purchase their services. This system is suitable when two criteria are met: (1) the relationship is voluntary and the patient can continue the relationship, end it, or change therapists as he wishes;

and (2) the patient can afford the high cost of the treatment, which may run as high as $10,000 a year for several years. Most who receive mental health services today do not meet these criteria. They are of moderate means or even poor.

Both private and public sectors will be discussed in this chapter. The emphasis will be on the public sector, for two reasons: (1) most individuals receive services from that sector, either because they initially cannot afford private services or because their personal resources have been drained before the private services became effective, and (2) the public sector employs most of the mental health and human service workers.

The Private Sector

The major mental health delivery system in the private sector is that of the private psychiatric hospital, sanitorium, and psychiatric ward of a general hospital. This system invariably occurs in the traditional medical model and is based on the doctor-patient relationship. Private hospitals and wards provide a back-up service for the private practitioner. If the private psychotherapist (usually an M.D.) feels the patient can no longer manage his daily life, he has the patient admitted to a private psychiatric hospital, either voluntarily or by commitment. The patient's original doctor usually remains in control of the case throughout the hospitalization, much as a family doctor controls a case in a medical hospital.

Usually there are two alternatives in the private hospital system: (1) the patient is admitted under third-party payment (health insurance) and is treated until he is cured or discharged but within a time period not exceeding 90 days (health insurance coverage for *mental diseases* usually does not exceed a 90-day period following admission); at the end of this period, the patient is sent home, no matter what his condition or he is transferred to a state mental hospital; (2) a family has sufficient money to be able to afford prolonged hospitalization, in which case the private hospital is willing to keep the patient until he is cured, even if the process takes years. It is not unusual for a 12-month hospitalization to cost $25,000 or more.

The major therapies in private hospitals are chemotherapy, electroconvulsive therapy, and one-to-one psychotherapy (between

127

therapist and patient), supplemented by activity therapy sessions in a hospital ward. The primary focus in the better-known hospitals (Menninger's Clinic, Chestnut Lodge) is the one-to-one, doctor-patient, verbal psychotherapy. In her popular book, *I Never Promised You a Rose Garden*, Hanna Green [1964] provides an excellent view of the private hospitalization of an adolescent girl. Miss Green describes the experiences of a 16-year-old schizophrenic girl during a three-year hospitalization and her relatively successful course in therapy.

The Public Sector

Public mental health delivery systems are big business. They include programs funded and operated by federal, state, and local governments and in some cases (such as many community mental health centers), programs partially or fully funded by charitable organizations. In 1970 state mental hospitals served over 338,592 patients, and in 1972 state mental health budgets totaled $3.2 billion. The addition of funds used to support public mental health clinics and Veterans Administration psychiatric hospitals brings the expenditure to a very high level. The following news item gives some idea of the magnitude of the problem:

MENTAL ILLNESS IN AMERICAN FAMILIES

Citing government statistics, a National Institute of Mental Health psychologist says that there is growing evidence that "almost no family in the nation is entirely free of mental disorders."

Dr. David Rosenthal suggested that the incidence of mental disorders may figure prominently among the causes of the country's social turbulence and disorders, including crime and racial unrest.

Based on the 1967 institute survey, Rosenthal concluded that possibly 60 million Americans are borderline schizophrenics or exhibit other deviant mental behavior in the schizophrenic category.

"Indeed," Rosenthal said in a report to the National Academy of Science, "it may very well be that the 'normal' person, with respect to mental health, does not represent a norm at all but rather an ideal—relatively rare—that most of us would like to achieve."

Rosenthal said there are more than 1.75 million schizophrenic persons walking the streets besides at least 500,000 in hospitals. Schizophrenia, one of the major mental illnesses, includes a tendency to withdraw from reality and often involves hallucinations and delusions.

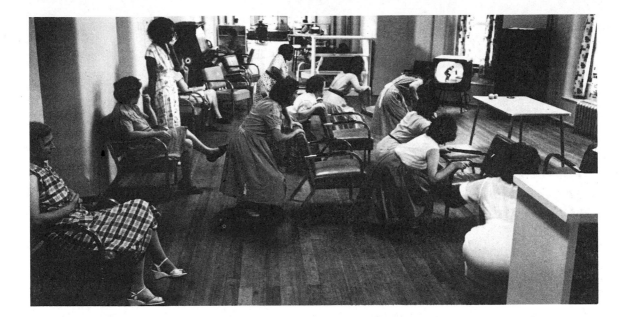

Two views of the inside of a state mental hospital. (Top,
photo by Inge Morath, courtesy Magnum; bottom,
photo by Bill Stanton, courtesy Magnum.)

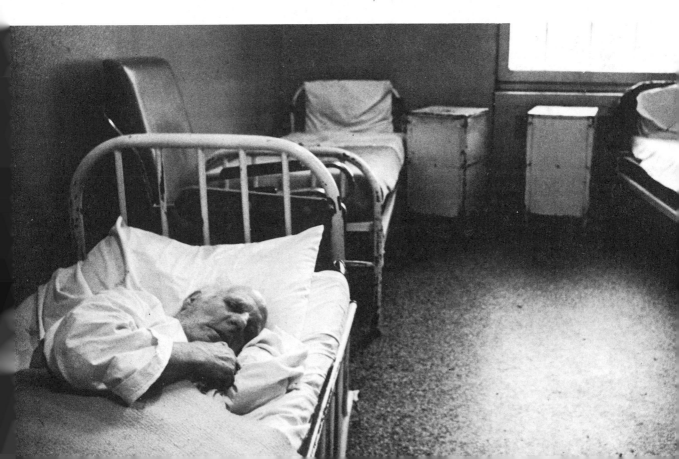

Rosenthal said other statistics from the survey indicate: 90,000 Americans were hospitalized in 1967 for depression and "many times more never found their way to a hospital." On suicide: "At least once every minute someone in the United States tries to kill himself, and once every 24 minutes the attempt is successful." "There are 9 million people in the United States with a serious drinking problem, or about one out of every 22 persons, whose annual cost to the nation is $10 billion."

Per patient, per day expenditures in public inpatient facilities average $18 to $20 a day, compared to $100 to $150 a day and up in private psychiatric hospitals. The relatively low levels of funding available, particularly in past years (in 1956 only an average of $3 per day per patient was allotted nationwide), has hampered the development of effective mental health delivery services.

Public services come under the two main categories of *outpatient* and *inpatient* mental health settings. Although some institutions provided both services within the same organization, until recently there were very few. These categories will be dealt with separately.

Outpatient Mental Health Settings

The outpatient category includes a variety of settings, the most common of which are mental health clinics and partial hospitalization, including day hospitals, night hospitals, and aftercare programs.

The Mental Health Clinic

The modern mental health clinic (or center) is an outgrowth of the mental hygiene movement of Adolf Meyer early in this century. Meyer was a psychiatrist who saw what he considered to be the far-reaching importance of providing alternatives to incarceration for behaviorally deviant persons.

Contemporary mental health clinics usually operate within the more or less traditional model. They employ professionals such as social workers, psychologists, and psychiatrists, but few *nonprofessionals*. They are usually directed by a psychiatrist though occasionally by a doctoral-level psychologist or master's-level social worker. Staff usually report to a supervisior in their own discipline;

in terms of *function*, they do not move freely from one discipline to another, with the exception that virtually all counsel patients.

In most clinics treatment consists of the one-to-one counseling, or psychotherapy, session. It is only within the last 5 to 10 years that any but the most progressive clinics have begun to experiment with group techniques. Because of this concentration on individual techniques, it is not unusual to encounter clinics which maintain three- to six-months waiting lists of patients who need service, a demand the clinics are unable to meet.

Characteristic of many clinics is selection of the patients they will treat. Most do not attempt to treat the disadvantaged patient, preferring, instead, to treat the white, middle-class, verbal, psychoneurotic patient. This is the area in which they have had their greatest success.

The Community Mental Health Act of 1963 precipitated a degree of change in the functioning of a significant number of community mental health centers. To be eligible for federal funds, many centers reorganized themselves so as to provide services to the high-risk patient (usually disadvantaged, relatively nonverbal, with a severe disorder). Clinics began to provide what were called the "five essential services" required for funding: inpatient services, outpatient services, partial hospitalization, 24-hour emergency services, and consultation and education. These five services, when supplemented by an additional five (diagnostic, rehabilitative, precare and after care, training, and research and evaluation), were considered to represent a comprehensive approach to community mental health care.

While many worthwhile changes have appeared because of the 1963 legislation, serious questions have arisen about the effectiveness of these modified mental health clinic programs. Some experts consider the 1963 act the first major battle to be mounted against the dominant medical model in mental health services. It was a battle that was lost, however, because the result was a transfer of the medical model (which had been so dominant in inpatient psychiatric hospitals) to the community mental health center. An excellent investigation of the community mental health center system has recently been completed by Franklin Chu and Sharland Trotter [1972] under the leadership of consumer advocate Ralph Nader.

Partial Hospitalization Settings

The main function of partial hospitalization is to provide an intensive program for behaviorally disturbed persons who do not require residential care. It includes day hospital, night hospital, and aftercare programs. Staff patterns closely correspond to the clinic's setting, use of professionals, as well as activity therapists and occupational therapists.

Treatment generally consists of chemotherapy. There is a heavy investment in group and individual psychotherapy, supplemented by organized activity sessions. The following schedule for a patient is typical of a weekday in a day-hospital program:

9:00 A.M.   Group psychotherapy
10:45   Expressive arts
12:00   Lunch
1:00 P.M.   Individual counseling session
2:45-4:00   Occupational therapy

Many programs include special therapy, depending on the expertise and personal interests of the staff. Examples are psychodrama, family therapy encounter groups, transactional analysis groups, and music therapy.

The major differences among the three types of services are structural rather than programmatic. The day hospital is intended to provide services to unemployed persons and housewives during the day, allowing them to return home to their families at night. The night hospital usually provides services from 6 to 10 P.M. and is oriented toward those who work during the day and who prefer to maintain their own residences. Aftercare programs are for patients recently discharged from a residential institution; they may have scheduling that includes day and evening hours. The focus of the aftercare program is on easing the transition back to *normal* life and preventing rehospitalization.

Inpatient Mental Health Settings

There are two major providers of inpatient mental health services in the public sector—the state and federal governments. State governments have provided inpatient services since the time of the American Revolution, beginning with the Pennsylvania Hospital. In terms of delivery of services to large numbers of patients, however, the federal government is a newcomer with the creation of the Veterans Administration. As is indicated in Chapter 5, inpatient mental health settings in the public sector (and incidentally, also in the private sector) have a long history of exclusion and extrusion of patients. For a variety of reasons, these institutions have been built in what were originally rural areas of the states. It seems that city-dwellers have almost deliberately banished the deviant to a distant, isolated place. Many of those mental institutions now in urban areas were originally in the country; the cities have simply grown up around them. Public institutions have only recently begun to overcome their past and to be able to provide less custodial and more meaningful services.

The State Mental Hospital

The traditional state mental hospital may be one of the most visible of the mental health delivery systems. Usually in a rural area, it often has an extensive "campus" surrounded by a high wrought iron fence enclosing old red brick buildings, one or more of which may have a large, ornate dome. Other similarities occur—a large patient population and inadequate staffing are common. Most states demand by law that the director be a medical doctor. As we saw earlier, most such hospitals are usually organized according to a departmental model.

The hospital usually has a heavily staffed admissions program which evaluates patients and decides what other program the patient should be transfered to for treatment. The hospital typically has several specialized programs—or units—often consisting of geriatrics, children's, and alcoholism programs, but the main focus is on the adult male and female patient, since this is the largest category of patients.

The major part of a *good* adult treatment program are chemotherapy, milieu therapy, group therapy, individual counseling, and activity therapy. Frequently there is a central rehabilitation workshop where patients receive training and experience in work skills, with or without salary. Many institutions still maintain pro-

133

grams designated as *industrial therapy*, in which patients work for the institution as dietary helpers, housekeepers, bakers, laundry workers, and so forth—without pay. The institutions often claim they cannot function without this unpaid labor.

Programs are often run by interdisciplinary teams composed of a physician, psychologist, nurse, social worker, activity therapist, and several psychiatric aides or attendants. Decisions are often made by group consensus, but in matters such as discharge, the physician usually has the final authority.

The patients come from the lower socioeconomic levels, are not articulate, and tend to exhibit the most severe behavioral disorders. By the time the patient reaches this last stop in his career as a patient, all other possibilities have been exhausted. The most severely disturbed usually end up in the least resourceful of the hospital's wards. Due to lack of techniques for dealing with the problems, the length of their stay tends to be long, usually years.

These trends are beginning to change. Because of increasing staff size and changes in attitudes about who should be incarcerated, patient populations have begun to decline. In state hospitals the inpatient population has decreased from a high of over 550,000 in 1955 to around 300,000 today.

Veterans Administration Psychiatric Services

In contrast to the resource-poor state mental hospital systems, the more recently developed Veterans Administration (V.A.) psychiatric system is financially well endowed. At a time when daily per-patient costs in state systems average $6 to $9, the federal V.A. costs per patient per day average $26.

Veterans Administration psychiatric services include both inpatient and outpatient systems, with the inpatient services being by far the most extensive. The services (which are provided only to those who have served in the military) are available through a large network of facilities across the country.

Many types of treatment in the V.A. hospitals parallel those in other institutions, but there tends to be a wider variety of regular treatment. In addition, the staff delivering the services often have better credentials. This is due to the higher salaries paid by the V.A., their higher standards, and their greater emphasis on the total cre-

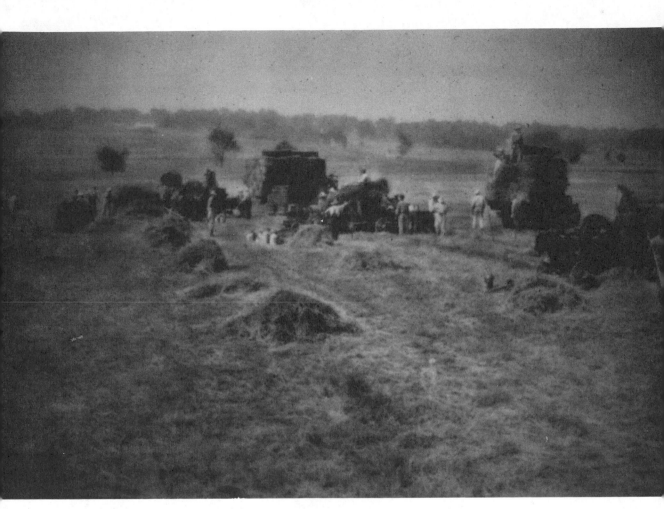

Institutional work therapy was and is common in State
hospitals. This picture from the 1930s illustrates the
unpaid labor provided by the "residents."

dentialing process common to the medical model (which is entrenched in the V.A. system).

The Veterans Administration, while open to the introduction of innovative treatments, seems unlikely to change its organization significantly so as to include large numbers of the new type of human service worker. The recent V.A. interest in the concept of self-help groups and other nontraditional programs, however, holds promise.

Neotraditional Mental Health Systems

A number of mental health systems exist which fit neither the traditional nor the human service models. While they are often based on a sprinkling of traditional concepts, they use the concepts nontraditionally. There may even be some question as to whether the term *mental health* should be applied to them; *neotraditional* (new-traditional) will have to do. The earliest of these systems were developed in response to problems which respond poorly to traditional treatment techniques, notably chronic recidivist psychotic disturbances and alcoholism. Drug abuse problems were included later.

The neotraditional systems tend to reject the involvement of professionals (with credentials) as therapists but rather turn to the use of individuals who have themselves surmounted the problem. Alcoholics Anonymous, Synanon, and Recovery, Inc. are examples.

Alcoholics Anonymous

Alcholics Anonymous has banded together in a formal self-help system. It features a 13-step program, with the goal of achieving sobriety. The program includes weekly meetings at which all members confess to the others that they are alcoholics, and in intimate detail recount their transgressions. A major requirement of belonging to the group is complete devotion to helping each other stay sober. Any member may call another at any hour for moral and physical support. The organization seems to have had remarkable success, perhaps due to the immense emotional and psychological investment made by the members.

Synanon

Synanon is the prototype of self-help drug-abuse programs. It is run by former addicts very much on the order of a modern-day commune. Members live and work together in a mutually supportive arrangement, rejecting *professional* interference. Heavy emphasis is placed on what some people consider an almost brutally confrontative approach to lack of *self-honesty*. Synanon seems to have become a way of life for many ex-addicts and enjoys a high rate of success.

Recovery, Inc.

Based on the psychiatric theories of Abraham Low, who was once a professor of psychiatry at the University of Illinois Medical School, Recovery, Inc., since Low's death, has become consumer-funded and operated. Recovery, Inc.'s full title is The Association of Nervous and Former Mental Patients. It focuses on the use of willpower in avoiding deviant behavior.

Summary

There are numerous mental health delivery systems that continue to operate traditionally. Those described in this chapter are the major delivery systems which the human service worker will encounter in the field. By far the greatest expenditure of time, effort, and money is made in the public sector, even though the percapita expenditures remain small. In some instances, there seems to be progress in the direction of a human services network, but much remains to be done before that goal is reached.

Chapter 9 *The Traditional Technologies*

A major facet of the traditional mental health model is its investment in developing and using specific technologies for treating deviants. This investment may well be a reflection of today's broad reliance on technological solutions to social problems.

The medical model, in particular, has applied technology to the mental health field. Recent medical advances have been a direct result of scientific and technological advances. Medicine's reliance on technology carries an important message for mental health: if man can find the *right* technology, surely mental illness can be cured, whether chemically, surgically, eugenically, or psychologically.

This message is evident in the traditional mental health model through the proliferation of technologies aimed at curing, or at least changing, the behavior of those who are mentally ill, psychotic, or merely neurotic. Many of these technologies are effective to some degree, but none has produced the much-desired cure. At the very least, the beginning human service worker needs an introduction to today's major technologies, which we will attempt to provide in this chapter.

The Somatic Therapies

The major somatic therapies are chemotherapy, the convulsive therapies, and psychosurgery. These therapies are the exclusive province of the physican, since they most closely resemble actual medical techniques.

As was discussed in Chapter 5, *somatic therapies* predate recorded history. Even relatively recent somatic therapies seem strange in retrospect. For example, hydrotherapy, which was common in the 1950s seems in the 1970s almost medieval.

Hydrotherapy involves wrapping patients in *wet packs* which alter their body temperature and limit their body movements, which it was thought, would have a tranquilizing effect. The development of the technique brought into existence special wards to which *acting-out* patients could be transferred. Unfortunately the wards were used to threaten patients as a means of controlling them. In many hospitals the warning "you'll be transferred to hydro" became a genuine threat. With the advent of chemotherapies (a much more effective tranquilizing technique), the use of hydrotherapy gradually declined.

Chemotherapy

Although a number of chemotherapies such as the bromides have been used for years, the introduction of the phenothiazine chlorpromazine in the early 1950s marked the beginning of their wide usage. These chemicals have the effect of modifying affective states without massively decreasing cognitive functioning. Since a variety of chemicals are used, our discussion in this chapter will be limited to those most commonly used.

The action of the chemicals remains something of a mystery, but it is believed that the phenothiazines decrease the action of the neurotransmitter, while the iminodibenzyls increase the action. Therefore the phenothiazines deplete (or inactivate) norepinephrine

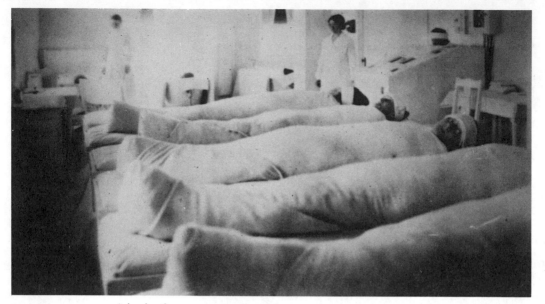

A hydrotherapy program, using wet packs in a state
hospital during the 1930s and 40s. Similar treatment was
still common in the early 1960's.

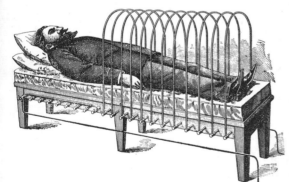

An example of early electrotherapy (1895).
(Courtesy New York Public Library.)

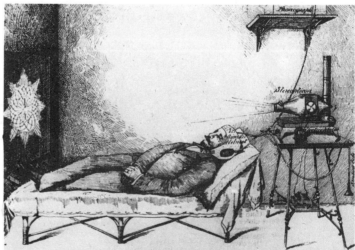

Dr. Corning's audio-visual tranquilizer used in treating
the depressed with music and lantern slides. The patient
is placed on a low divan and an acoustic hood is
applied. The harmonic vibrations and pictures of
"enchanting beauty" were supposed to give the patient
a "new somberness." (Courtesy The Bettmann Archive.)

in the brain, which usually produces a sedative, or depressive, action; the iminodibenzyls increase (or activate) norepinephrine, producing an antidepressant effect. Most researchers admit that this rationale does not entirely explain the impressive effects of the chemicals on disturbed patients. They are used primarily because they seem to work. Following are descriptions of several of the major drugs.

Chlorpymazine hydrachloride. Commonly known by the brand name Thorazine, chlorpymazine may be administered orally or intramuscularly. Oral dosages usually do not have to be more than 800 milligrams a day, but dosages in institutions sometimes reach 1,200 to 4,000 mg. per day. When the patient is no longer disturbed, the dosage may be reduced. This drug has a tranquilizing effect on a variety of disturbances—tension, overactivity, agitation, destructiveness, and paranoid reactions. In the acute schizophrenic, hallucinations and delusions often disappear. In many cases patients become more amenable to psychotherapy. Persistent delusions and hallucinations are often no longer disturbing to the patient. The drug is not effective in all cases, but even with chronic patients, 50 to 60 percent have shown improvement. A major problem with chemotherapy, however, are the side effects. For example, chlorpymazine can cause heart palpitation, hypertension, skin reactions, jaundice, parkinsonism, and other side effects.

Thioridazin. Sold under the brand name Mellaril, this chemical produces clinical effect similar to that of Thorazine, but with fewer side effects. The usual daily dosage is 300 to 800 mg. in psychotic patients.

Imipramine. This iminodebenzyl derivative is marketed under the trade name, Tofranil. It is considered a highly effective antidepressant in dosages of 200 to 300 mg. per day. Tofranil seems most effective when used to combat the psychotic depression states rather than the neurotic depressive reaction. Its use usually results in a reduction of self-depreciation and self-accusation, followed by increased activity and socialization. Large doses may result in motor tremors and cardiovascular symptoms, however.

Amitriptyline. Sold under the name Elavil, this drug has an action similar to Tofranil, with less side effects likely. It also has a hypnotic action, which makes it useful for patients suffering from sleep disturbance.

141

There is some controversy over the use of such chemical restraints as these on individuals who have little or no choice as to whether they will receive the drugs. The impressive effectiveness of the drugs so far, though, seem to insure their use for some time to come.

The Convulsive Therapies

The convulsive therapies have been in use for over 40 years, but to date there has been no satisfactory explanation of why they work. Their use is justified on a purely empirical basis (again, *because they work*).

Electroconvulsive Therapy

The introduction of electroconvulsive therapy (ECT) by Ugo Cerletti is described in Chapter 5. The technique consists of lightly restraining the patient on a horizontal mat, placing a padded tongue depressor between his teeth, applying electrodes to both sides of his forehead, and administering 79 to 130 volts of alternating current for 0.1 to 0.5 seconds. The patient instantly becomes unconscious and experiences approximately 10 seconds of tonic and 15 seconds of clonic convulsion. Treatment is usually given three times a week for up to 30 treatments. ECT seems particularly effective in the treatment of *involutional melancholia* and the depressive phase of manic-depressives. It is claimed that recovery is possible in 80 percent of the cases. The ECT seems to relieve depressive feelings, quiet the patient, and promote socialization. It is useful in the treatment of acute schizophrenia, when affective or emotional features are present, by promoting a lessening of the patient's symptoms.

Complications can occur, including memory loss, ranging from a tendency to forget names to severe confusion. Memory loss may last as long as several months. Fractures and dislocations of bones occur in about 20 percent of the patients treated, but death is extremely rare.

Insulin Shock Treatment

The original reports on the effect of insulin shock treatment on excited schizophrenics were published in the early 1930s, and the basic technique has changed little since then. The injection of insulin reduces the sugar content of the blood, which interferes with the oxidation processes of brain cells, thus preventing proper metabolism and leading to coma. Insulin shock treatment (IST) is relatively drastic. It is critically important that patients be in good physical health before it is attempted.

The standard technique is to inject 15 to 25 units of insulin, which is increased by 10 to 15 units daily until the required depth of coma is reached. This process usually takes 7 to 15 treatments. Because of the danger of severe complications, intensive 24-hour nursing supervision is required. The coma is terminated by the administration of carbohydrates. Treatment usually continues until the patient has experienced 50 hours of coma.

The use of IST is limited (and works best with) acute schizophrenics. There is an inverse relationship between length of illness and effectiveness of treatment. Its effect, when successfully used, is to reduce schizophrenic symptoms.

IST may be dangerous and can be fatal; in spite of all precautions, there is a mortality rate of 0.5 to 1 percent. Prolonged comas sometimes occur, which may lead to permanent brain damage. There are two types of convulsions: *early* and *late.* The early type (grand mal) is fairly easily controlled, but the late type is an indication of failure and usually results in death or irreversible coma. Because of the possibly disastrous side effects, IST is no longer a treatment of choice; but one does occasionally hear of its use.

Psychosurgery

The historical development of psychosurgery is briefly discussed in Chapter 5. Basically it is a surgical technique consisting of entering the brain case by various methods and cutting the nerve fibers connecting the thalamus and frontal lobe. The patient first becomes stuporous or confused. He doesn't care about his surroundings; he may become incontinent; he must be fed; and he may become agitated and destructive. During the first few weeks after the operation the patient must be retrained in the social controls he has lost.

In successful cases, patients who have shown anxiety and agita-

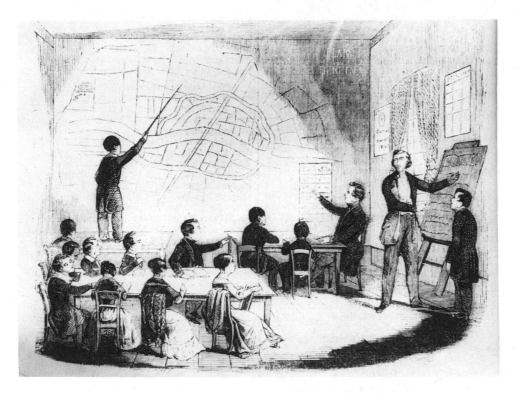

Early application of occupational therapy. Above, Dr.
Segert's Institution in Leipzig, Germany. Below,
vocational training in an English asylum about 1860.
(Above courtesy The Bettmann Archive; below courtesy
New York Public Library.)

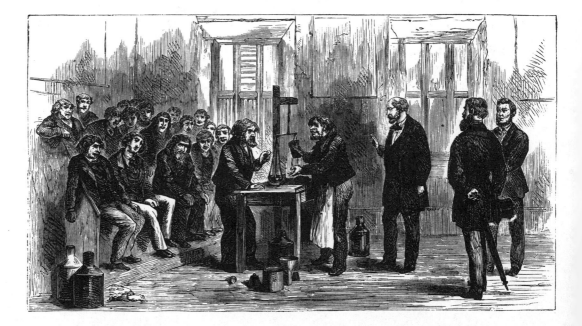

tion, depression, aggressiveness, hostility, and extremely impulsive behavior may become quiet and well behaved. Psychosurgery—or lobotomy—is most successful with acute schizophrenics and schizophrenics who have manifested disturbance for less than two years. Because of the rather extensive consequences, however, it is recommended only as a last resort. In addition to the quieting effects of the surgery, patients may sometimes be reduced to lethargy, they may sometimes have accentuated and unpleasant personality traits, become facetious or act childishly, be unable to manage their own financial and social affairs, be irresponsible, lack sensitivity, have shallow emotional responses, be tactless, lack imagination, be lazy, vulgar, and profane.

Because of these many side effects, the use of psychosurgery has declined since the 1950s, but in the early 1970s, there has been a resurgence in some parts of the country, particularly in an attempt to control children with behavioral problems. This resurgence includes the use of a number of new techniques, including lasers and cryosurgery (the use of supercold liquids to destroy cell tissues). But there continues to be significant opposition to these techniques.

The Psychotherapies

The psychotherapies are without doubt the major mental health technique of this century. To the layman they may well have become *the* technique, due partly to a preoccupation with them in literature and movies. In the past 50 years, there have been a proliferation of basic types of therapies. For purposes of illustration, we will focus here on two basic theories of psychotherapy, psychoanalytic and Rogerian.

The definition of *traditional psychotherapy* depends on the psychotherapeutic theory one has in mind, but there are several features common to most. When the following criteria are met, there is fairly common agreement on calling the resultant process *psychotherapy:*

1. A relatively durable interpersonal relationship exists between two or more persons.

2. At least one of the participants has special experience, training, or education in interpersonal relationships.

145

3. At least one of the participants has entered into the relationship because of dissatisfaction with his interpersonal or emotional adjustment, or in the case of institutional settings, has entered into the relationship on the basis of the opinion of others.

4. The method used is a psychological one.

5. The procedure is based on a theory of mental disorder and the individual disorder of the patient.

6. The goal is an eventual solution to the problems as defined by the therapist or the patient.

Psychotherapy usually aims at the progress of the recipient toward normality, maturity, increased competence, and self-actualization (living up to one's potential). Although the goals are similar, the techniques vary.

Psychoanalytic Psychotherapy

Most psychotherapeutic theories are complex systems which require lengthy study for useful understanding, and psychoanalysis is perhaps the most complex of all the psychotherapeutic theories. One of its basic concepts is that there are fixed stages of development which an organism must pass through successfully in order to mature correctly. The human organism originally functions on the basis of the *pleasure principle,* insisting on immediate gratification of its needs. These inborn forces are called the *id,* the core of the unconscious mind. The developmental stages have been named according to the bodily zones that are energized by *libido* (life forces) operating on the pleasure principle during that stage. For example, the oral stage is that period of life when the pleasure principle is gratified through the mouth. (In Freudian terms, the mouth is *erogenized.*) Each stage of development has certain crucial issues which must be resolved. If they are not, the individual may become fixed at that level of development, with attendant feelings and emotions repressed into the unconscious portion of his mind. In later life, stressful situations may precipitate distorted behavior which was once gratifying.

Psychoanalysis focuses on resurrecting these now unconscious feelings and emotions, which are assumed to be the prime motivators of behavior, assisting the individual to *work them*

146

through. A patient in the analytic session *free associates;* he talks about whatever comes to mind. The therapist notes what is said, as well as what may be behind what is said. At appropriate points the therapist interprets the *true* meaning of the patient's thoughts. It is believed that during the course of analysis a *transference reaction* takes place: the patient relives his early interpersonal conflicts, transferring them now to the therapist. The pathological effects of the earlier experiences are rectified by exposing the patient to these same emotional experiences, with the difference now being that the therapist maintains a different attitude from that of the parents originally. The therapist is objective and understanding; the patient is free to express his original feelings (as nearly as he can remember them)—whether fear, rage, anger—more honestly; he may also recognize that his reactions are no longer adequate. He can now change.

Rogerian or Patient-Centered Psychotherapy

The Rogerian psychotherapy techinque was developed by Carl Rogers, a psychologist originally at the University of Chicago. It is an outgrowth of a major school of personality theories which focus on self-concepts. Rogers' theories are based on the concept of the *phenomenal self,* the self-image a person experiences based on the sensory evidence he receives. This image does not necessarily correspond to reality and may not be the image the person would like to have.

Personality maladjustment is the result of an individual's inability to integrate all of his experiences, feelings, and desires into his phenomenal self. Each tries to perceive experiences and behave in ways that are consistent with this self-image. When he is confronted with new experiences or feelings that are inconsistent with his image of himself, he can either perceive them clearly and integrate them or deny and distort them. Maladjustment consists of perceiving inconsistent experiences, or feelings, as a threat, denying them to the consciousness, and thereby widening the gap between the phenomenal self and reality. Anxiety and tension result from this discrepancy between self-image and reality. Adjustment consists of having a self-image that is flexible and consistent with reality or that is able to change as new experiences occur.

The therapist's primary goal is to show warmth toward the patient and total acceptance of him, in order to provide a nonthreatening atmosphere in which the patient is able to explore his thoughts and feelings, including those he has previously denied, with no fear of censure. The therapist *never* criticizes, condemns, or judges. Within the confines of this relationship, the patient is expected to become able to resolve the conflicts between his phenomenal self and his reality.

The patient-centered therapy we are discussing is also known as *nondirective therapy*. Here the implication is that the therapist is less *directive* than the therapist in psychoanalysis and other similar therapies. There is less interpretation of what the patient does or says, for example. This approach, which puts the primary responsibility for change on the patient, relies heavily on the patient's growth and adjustment.

According to Rogers, there are five steps in psychotherapy:

1. *Opening phase*. The patient experiences psychological problems and actively seeks help.

2. *Expression and acceptance of feeling*. The therapist encourages the open expression of feelings, including those which in the past have been denied. He accepts and clarifies the feelings underlying the problems so that the patient can accept them as part of himself.

3. *Insight development*. The increased understanding and acceptance of the self leads to the development of insight:
(a) recognition and emotional acceptance of the real attitudes and desires of the self; (b) a clearer understanding of the causes behind one's behavior; (c) a fresh perception of the life situation (a new frame of reference); (d) clarification of the decisions that must be made and the possible courses of action.

4. *Positive steps*. As therapy progresses the patient begins to consider taking positive action (make decisions, change his behavior, and so on), which is clarified by the therapist.

5. *Termination*. As the patient becomes increasingly self-confident and integrated, there is less need for therapy. The termination decision is made by the patient as a step toward independence.

In nondirective, patient-centered Rogerian therapy, the patient is allowed to proceed at his own rate and in his own direction. There are no confrontations by the therapist and his role is one of acceptance, reflection, and classification of feelings.

Group Psychotherapy

Group psychotherapy is a series of variations on the basic theories of psychotherapy. There are a number of group psychotherapies, each based on a psychotherapeutic theory. For example, there is psychoanalytic group psychotherapy, nondirective group psychotherapy, Adlerian group psychotherapy and a host of others.

The major difference between group psychotherapy and the original psychotherapies is that in group psychotherapy, there is more than one patient in a session with one or more therapists. Usually two therapists and 7 to 10 patients attend the same session. The development of group psychotherapy is an outgrowth of the desire to provide a microculture for the patients and to increase the efficiency of the psychotherapeutic model.

The most important aspect of group psychotherapy is that it more closely resembles real-life situations and social relationships than does individual psychotherapy. In individual psychotherapy, everything is channeled from the patient to the therapist and back again, while in group psychotherapy, there are usually two therapists and a number of patients to provide feedback services with each other. Thus a variety of responses and reactions are available for the behavior displayed in the group setting. Most groups move through three broad phases of development: (1) group unification and development of identity, (2) group interaction and the observation of dynamics, and (3) resolution of dynamics and production of insights.

During group sessions, members may examine their pattern of relating to each other and to authority figures, as well as their behavior, motivation, and reactions to each other—all in a supportive atmosphere.

Many therapists prefer group psychotherapy to individual psychotherapy, feeling that it is effective or more effective than the familiar one-to-one therapy. It has the added value of economy, which may account for its widespread adoption in institutions. During a time when an individual therapist can see only one or two patients, a group therapist can see as many as 10. This efficiency is reflected in costs for private sessions; the cost of a private, individual

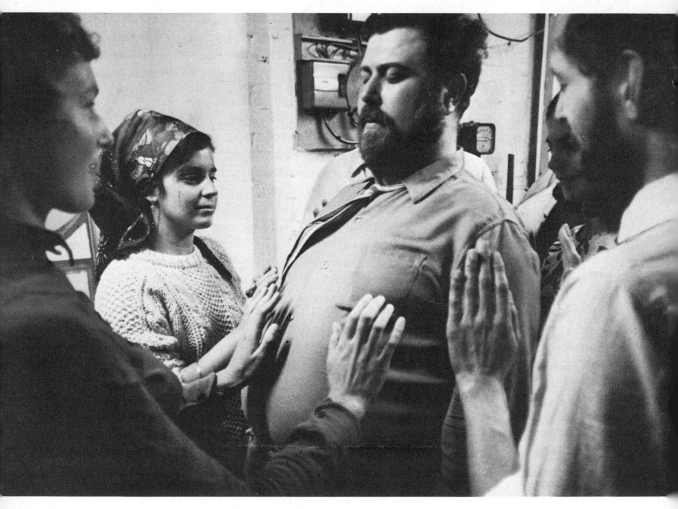

A recent development is the sensitivity group, a form of group psychotherapy. (Photo by Ian Berry, courtesy Magnum.)

session ranges from $25 to $50 an hour, while a private group session averages $7 to $10 an hour.

Family Therapy

Family therapy is a recent technique. It is based on the traditional mental health model and is an outgrowth of dissatisfaction with both individual and group psychotherapies. For years therapists have been concerned about the problem of lack of involvement or inappropriate involvement of family members in the therapy of the patient. Families were seen as not caring about the treatment their relatives were receiving or as interferring in it. For these reasons and for the reason that family members (parents and siblings) were felt to be primary in the development of psychological problems, a number of therapists began seeing entire families at a time in situations resembling group psychotherapy.

In this system the family is the main unit; it provides for the growth and maturation of its members. If the family transactions are disturbed, its members are likely to manifest behavior disorders that are symptomatic of the disturbance of the family unit. A major problem for the family unit is the tolerance of differences. The healthy family is able to tolerate differences among its members and to successfully work through the conflicts that result from these differences. The maladjusted family unit experiences individual differences as threats to its unity, and the ensuing conflicts lead to splits, coalitions, and scapegoating. Frequently, the *sick* member, who is initiallly identified as the patient, makes his adjustment to deviance in an abortive attempt to maintain the family unit. A number of cases have been reported of families in which, when one sick member dropped his deviant behavior, another member became disturbed—a role exchange.

The major objective of family therapy is the reestablishing of rational communication between family members, communication that will correct the distorted relationships which contribute to the family problem or problems. Family therapy allows the family to reassess and reorganize its alliances and resolve to accept the real or imagined differences between its members.

151

The Family As A Patient

In almost all traditional psychotherapies, the patient meets alone with his therapist and is expected to tell no one—not even his closest relatives—what goes on in the sessions. A contrast to this is family therapy. Several relatives, spanning two or three generations, see their psychotherapist together for treatment. The therapy does not always probe as deeply as individual therapy does, but it costs less in time and money.

Of the 1,000 or so psychiatrists, psychologists, and workers in the United States who practice family therapy, one of the most innovative is psychiatrist Norman Paul (Bourne and Ekstrand [1973]) who believes that family troubles frequently are caused not by a generation gap but by a *communication* gap, which family members can bridge by sharing their innermost feelings with each other. In one case Paul reports, a 39-year-old journalist named Lewis, about to divorce his wife to marry a young girl, had broken down in sobs as he recalled his grief over the death of his beloved Aunt Anna.

"She was always accepting me as I am. Being with her was like peace," Lewis said. Reviewing his childhood sorrow as his wife listened, he recognized that his girl friend represented the goal of his lifelong search for another Aunt Anna. This led him to return to his wife, who was now more understanding because she had shared his secret feelings.

Since that time, Paul has used the Lewis tape to diagnose hidden, crippling grief in other families. A brusque father whose son William was having emotional trouble got "a feeling of being half lost" when he heard Lewis' sobs. Then, said Paul, "he recollected the time when he himself had felt intense grief"—when his father remarried. Paul helped the father reconstruct what he knew but had blocked off: that when he was four his mother had killed both his nine-month-old sister and herself. Because he had repressed sorrow instead of facing it, he had never recovered from the experience. Under Paul's guidance he saw that he was jealous because his son still had what he himself had lost so early—a mother. It soon became clear that that jealousy was the real cause of the boy's emotional disturbance.

When divorce threatens to split a family, Paul often uses the *freeze-split* technique. He advises husband and wife to live apart for awhile, in order to find out what emotional problems left over from their premarriage days remain to be solved. In one instance a woman who nearly broke up her marriage—by beginning a series of affairs just as her daughter turned four—revealed in therapy that she had lost her mother when she herself was four. To Paul, the conclusion was inescapable: the first affair "was an attempt to remove herself from her daughter just as her own mother had left her."

The reward for facing the reality of envy and other painful emotions during family therapy, Paul concludes, is "a sense of oneself, a sense of self-esteem and expectant mastery over whatever might be coming down the pike."

An important difference between family therapy and group psychotherapy is that in family therapy the participants enter the situation with a long-standing system of roles and interactions and probably will leave still linked together by their familial ties but with the beginnings of change. The usual group psychotherapy relationship dates from the first session; the therapist need not be concerned with what went before in the group's interrelationships, since they don't apply.

Evaluation

It is disconcerting to realize that little hard evidence exists which demonstrates that either somatic or psychological therapies have an identifiable therapeutic effect. A search of the literature yields this conclusion: for practically every published article that purports to show the effectiveness of a particular therapy, another can be found that indicates the therapy does not work. This brings the traditional mental health field to about where it began: relying on long-standing beliefs, assumptions, and theories.

It may be incomprehensible to you that so many unproven techniques are the treatment of choice in spite of evidence in some cases of long-lasting, damaging side effects (especially with somatic techniques). This is related to the patients' need that their professionals be experts. This situation is compounded by the fact that the patients and the public want an easy answer—a pill, an injection, a *treatment*.

Since many concepts of the traditional mental health field remain questionable because of the lack of definitive research and evaluation, the human service worker is in the position of having to make his own decisions on the basis of the merits and efficacy of various treatments. In the course of his studies, he will encounter conflicting reports, which will make his decision-making all the more difficult.

As a final note on the evaluation of the therapies, we would like to mention an interesting concept. The concept has been called the *one-third phenomenon* and can be summarized as follows: surveys of the literature on the therapies indicate that no matter *what* the treatment (or even whether there is any treatment), at any given time, one-third of those persons expressing *behavioral deviance* (broadly defined) eventually improve to a considerable degree, one-third improve slightly, and one-third do not improve at all. The question of why, how and under what circumstances remains unanswered.

Summary

The development of specific techniques has been a major characteristic of the traditional model. Most technologies have been used widely in spite of a lack of understanding as to *why* they work or even how well they work. The continued use of particular techniques seems to depend more on the beliefs and assumptions of the practioners than on hard data supporting their effectiveness.

Chapter 10 *The Traditional Professions: Role, Function, and Training*

The essence of the traditional mental health model is transmitted mainly by the professionals who operate within it. In a very real sense, they transmit a particular set of cultural values. Over the years their function has been fragmented through specialization into various roles which have evolved into "professions," with each profession laying claim to a particular facet of the deviant individual. By and large, each profession respects the other's specialty. In some cases, they have gone so far as to lobby for legislation designed to protect their function by law from encroachment by other professions. Recently psychiatrists and psychoanalysts opposed psychologists over the issue of third-party payments (insurance and Medicare-Medicaid) for psychotherapy. The medical profession attempted to limit third-party payment for psychotherapy to medical professionals while at the same time excluding psychologists.

The traditional professions, however, have more in common with each other than with the new human service worker. Tending to accept their respective roles, they disagree only as to who can and cannot engage in the more broadly defined mental health services such as psychotherapy and administration. But at least there is common agreement on the basic definition of the professions.

In this chapter we will look at the role of the major traditional mental health professions as they are defined today. These professions—psychiatrist, psychoanalyst, psychologist, social worker, nurse, rehabilitation counselor, activity therapist, psychiatric aide—in some agencies work as a team and in others as separate entities in the departmental service model.

Role and Function

The Psychiatrist and the Psychoanalyst

The psychiatrist is considered the dean of the mental health team. He is usually a member of the American Psychiatric Association. Following graduation from medical school, he completes an approved residency in psychiatry, often in a department of psychiatry in a hospital or clinic. His training and credentials give him the broadest and most comprehensive role.

The psychiatrist prescribes medication, makes diagnoses, develops treatment plans, administers somatic therapies such as electroconvulsive shock, engages in psychotherapy, and makes clinical or administrative decisions about patient discharges and privileges. Although much of his function has been taken over by other mental health professionals in various mental health systems, his primary function of medical practitioner is intact. His position as a medical doctor gives him power and authority and invests him with prestige.

The process of becoming a *psychiatrist* is lengthy and costly. From the time he enters medical school until he receives his certification as a psychiatrist is usually a minimum of five years and costs $20,000 to $35,000. To become a *psychoanalyst* takes at least three additional years and a 300-hour analysis—which costs an additional $20 to $30 thousand. These costs, however, are often supported by federal and state grants. The financial rewards can be substantial. Table 10.1,

Table 10.1
Average Gross Income of Psychiatrists and Psychoanalysts

Income	Psychiatrists	Psychoanalysts
	Number=127 (percent)	Number=33 (percent)
Under 15,000	12	0
15,000-19,999	13	6
20,000-24,999	23	9
25,000-29,999	17	3
30,000-39,999	18	21
40,000-49,999	10	33
50,000-59,999	6	24
60,000-69,999	1	3
70,000 and over	0	3

from Arnold R. Rogow's book, *The Psychiatrists* [1970], presents conservative figures for psychiatrists and psychoanalysts, based on a small but representative sample.

In this sample, 35 percent of the psychiatrists earn over $30,000 a year, while 84 percent of the psychoanalysts earn over $30,000. That more psychoanalysts earn over $30,000 a year than do psychiatrists is explained partly by the fact that more psychiatrists are employed in public institutions, where the salaries are lower, while psychoanalysts are more likely to be engaged in lucrative private practice.

The Psychologist

Although the psychologists' national organization, the American Psychological Association, usually defines a *psychologist* as one who has earned a doctorate in philosophy (Ph.D.) in the study of psychology, many agencies employ psychologists who have a master's degree or less. After receiving his bachelor's degree, a psychologist usually takes three or four additional years of graduate study in psychology to obtain his doctorate. The cost of this education ranges from $5,000 to $15,000, depending on the school.

The education of the psychologist differs from that of the psychiatrist, in that psychology tends to be more theory- and research-oriented, with usually a one-year internship, while the psychiatrist's training tends to focus on a long residency which minimizes classroom training and maximizes practical experience.

The psychologist's original role in the mental health field was that of an evaluator. It was his job to measure the assets and liabilities of the patient, using what are known as psychometric techniques—tests such as the Rorschach, Thematic Apperception Test, Wechsler Adult Intelligence Scale, and the Stanford-Binet Intelligence Test.

In the past two decades psychologists have dramatically expanded their role to include that of *psychotherapist*. In most states they are allowed to practice private psychotherapy for a fee and to function as clinicians in state and federal agencies. In other words, they may work exactly as psychiatrists in all but purely medical positions.

In terms of income, psychologists remain second to psychiatrists. While some have high incomes, most do not approach those of the average psychiatrist, much less the psychoanalyst's. The average salary for a psychologist in the Veterans Administration is about $18,000 a year. In state institutions, it is considerably less.

The Social Worker

The professional *social worker* usually has a master's degree in social work (M.S.W.). There are few of them in public institutions, however. The social worker's traditional role has been to work with the patient on his social history, development, family relationships, and socioeconomic problems. In the traditional institution, the social worker's role corresponds to that of the family and friends: he counsels the family while the doctor treats the patient and makes living arrangements for the patient after he has been discharged.

The social worker's role has also broadened in recent years. Today, social workers engage in psychotherapy and group counseling, function as team members, and act as administrators. They function much as psychiatrists and psychologists do, but they cannot legally perform medical acts or ethically do psychometric testing.

Economically, most social workers are not as successful as

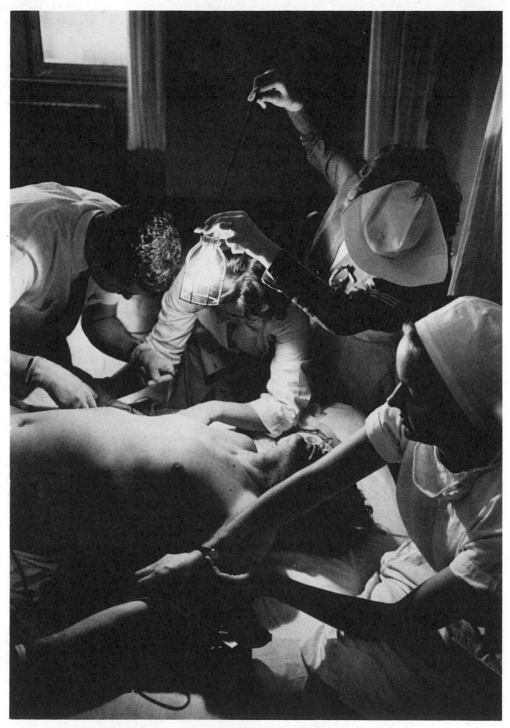

A crisis situation requiring a combination of traditional professionals. (Photo by Ian Berry, courtesy Magnum.)

psychiatrists or psychologists (the average social worker's annual salary is $9,000 to $14,000). There is a much smaller percentage of social workers in private practice than psychologists or psychiatrists.

The Nurse

Two types of *nurses* are easily distinguishable in the field of mental health—the psychiatric nurse, who has advanced training or a degree in psychiatric nursing, and the nurse who works in a psychiatric facility because it is nearby or because she has the interest while lacking the credentials of a psychiatric nurse. The credentialed psychiatric nurse is rare in public psychiatric facilities. Most registered nurses are employed in psychiatric institutions directly from nurses training or a general hospital after having completed a three- to six-months affiliation with a psychiatric hospital during their training.

Traditionally the nurse in a public psychiatric facility functioned in a role similar to that of the nurse in a general medical hospital. She gave medication, took temperatures, blood pressure, and pulse, and was concerned mainly with the maintenance operation of a ward. Her most important function was to alert the doctor to signs of *physical* illness in the patients.

Her role has changed considerably over the years. She may now counsel, participate in group therapy, act as a milieu therapist, and so on, the major limitation possibly being that she can function this way only *within an institution;* she is usually not certified to provide these services outside the institution she is employed in.

Salaries of registered nurses in public institutions vary. On the average, they range from approximately $7,000 to $10,000 a year.

The Rehabilitation Counselor

The *rehabilitation counselor* is usually certified with a master's degree in rehabilitation and vocational counseling. Many, however, with bachelor's degrees hold this title.

The typical master's-level counselor has taken a one- or two-year graduate program of study, focusing on the techniques of counseling the physically or mentally vocationally handicapped individual. He works in a central rehabilitation program, concentrating on verbally counseling patients about their feelings related to work abilities and actually *training* the handicapped person in activities relating to gainful employment. In some situations he is a member of a ward treatment team.

Rehabilitation counselor salaries are in the $7,000-$12,000 range.

The Activity Therapist

The certified *activity therapist* usually has a master's degree from an activity therapy graduate program of one or two years' duration. Most who work as activity therapists, however, do not have a graduate degree; they are activity therapists on the basis of a working title rather than credentials.

The activity therapist provides structured activity and recreational programs for patients (that have desirable therapeutic effects), which may include calisthenics, sports, games, dances, parties, and tours. The ideal activity therapy program includes a relationship between therapist and patient that will improve the patient's socialization capabilities.

As in the other professions in recent years, the role of the activity therapist has become blurred. Activity therapists are frequently team members; they participate in milieu and group therapy, and counsel patients, in addition to conducting activity therapy.

The activity therapist who lacks a master's degree is among the lowest paid of the professionals, earning on the average, $6,000 to $10,000 a year.

The Psychiatric Aide

The *psychiatric aide* is included in this list of traditional professionals despite the fact that most professionals would contend that he is "only a worker" and not really a professional. This discrimination is most likely based on the fact that one does not need a college degree to be a psychiatric aide. These individuals make up the greatest number of staff in most public institutions.

There are few qualifications for being a psychiatric aide or attendant. In most cases a person needs only a high school diploma,

161

and sometimes less. He is hired as a trainee and placed in a six-months training program where he is taught the basic routines he must follow. This program centers on nursing service-oriented activities and content, such as body structure and function, nursing skills, and medication.

The psychiatric aide usually does not function in a positive, therapeutic way; he operates as a repressive custodian. The line of authority ends with him. It is his responsibility to maintain a clean, quiet ward. He runs errands, deals with physically acting-out patients, cleans and dresses the incontinent, guards the door, and so on. In many cases, the aide's job description *forces* him to be custodial and repressive.

In recent years, there have been a number of attempts by institutions to use psychiatric aides as agents of change instead of as custodians. Francine Sobey [1970] has gathered data from over 185 government-sponsored mental health programs on this movement and published it in her book, *The Nonprofessional Revolution in Mental Health.*

The role of the psychiatric aide is changing perhaps more than that of any other mental health worker. In some cases salaries have kept pace with the change, in other cases, not. The psychiatric aide remains poorly paid, with an average salary ranging from $3,600 to $7,000 a year.

Psychiatric aides themselves have taken a major step to change their role function and identification with the creation of the National Association of Human Service Technologies, an organization which provides services similar to those of a *professional* organization: newsletter, conventions, statements on ethics, and so forth.

Training

The beliefs, assumptions, ideology, and philosophy of the traditional mental health model are transmitted from generation to generation of professionals by existing education and training. Individuals become members of a profession either by undergoing several years of graduate education or by intensive on-the-job training provided by experienced senior members of the profession.

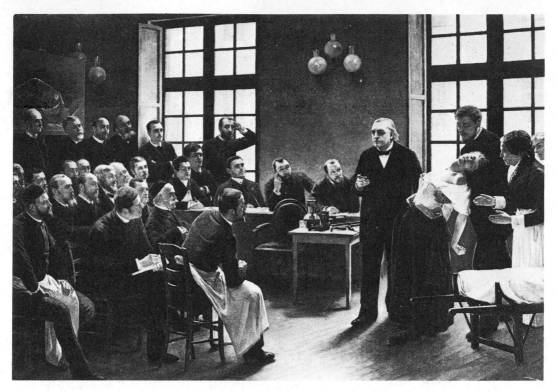

Part of the training of the traditional professionals —
a lecture by Jean Charcot at the Salpetrière. Freud was
one of Charcot's students. (Courtesy The
Bettmann Archive.)

Traditional treatment of a patient, 1892. (Courtesy New
York Public Library.)

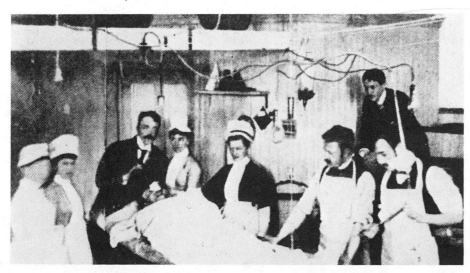

Most of the time, the person entering a field of study is highly receptive to the accumulated knowledge of his chosen field. He is usually young, motivated, and wants to learn about his chosen field. He tends to be uninformed about what it is really like. He believes his instructors are experts, for after all, they have years of experience. It is not surprising, then, that the newly graduated professional may be more of a traditionalist than those with experience. The new professional probably has received his training from an academician who, more likely than not, has not worked in a public institution recently.

An example of the discrepancy between graduate education and actual experience in clinical psychology will illustrate this point. Most clinical psychology programs place heavy emphasis on learning psychometric testing, yet there is little psychometric testing done by clinical psychologists today.

A second and more widespread example is the emphasis in most professional graduate programs on the theory and techniques relevant to neurosis psychopathology. In fact, however, most persons graduating from such programs will work in the public sector where they will deal with the most severely damaged deviants. Unfortunately, major deviancies receive the least amount of attention in most traditional graduate programs.

Traditional mental health graduate and training programs seem to be related to what *was* rather than what *is* or *should be*. Their focus in on *facts* discovered in the past rather than on questions that remain to be examined.

Summary

The traditional mental health professional—psychiatrist, psychoanalyst, psychologist, social worker, nurse, rehabilitation counselor, activity therapist, and psychiatric aide—is the transmitter of the traditional mental health model. He functions according to a basic, implicit agreement on the roles and areas of responsibility.

The basic tenets of the culture, the beliefs, assumptions, ideologies, and philosophies of the traditional mental health model are passed from generation to generation by the educational and training models. The 200-plus-year-old history of the model lends great impetus to its continued existence despite the many questions raised about its effectiveness and appropriateness.

Part III

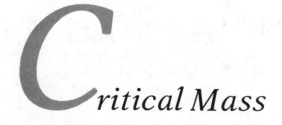

Critical Mass

Chapter 11 Expectations and Malfunctioning

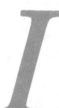n this chapter we will examine the expectations of the medical model, as well as its failure thus far to achieve those expectations.

Expectations of the Medical Model

The expectation that someone someday would discover a vaccine, a cure for mental illness was prevalent in the decades 1920-1950 when L.J. Meduna introduced Metrazol shock treatment, Manfred Sukel insulin shock therapy, Ugo Celeretti electric shock therapy, and Egas Moniz won the Nobel Prize for the development of lobotomy surgical techniques. Dr. Philip Bower, in a personal communication while chief psychologist of Elgin State Hospital, described the expectation well:

There was, for instance, the hope that substances related to psychiatric illnesses could be found in the bodies of the patients, that drugs could "cure," or that the "illness" could be so well understood and documented by an elite group of intellectuals that therapy could be prescribed precisely. The emphasis was on investigation with hope of future solution, and perhaps there was a Golden Age of Investigation of "mental illness". . . .

Persons thought to be mentally ill came or were brought to trained professionals for examination and diagnosis. The psychiatrist then prescribed what he considered appropriate treatment. It was an illusion that has dominated the thinking of mental health workers ever since.

In the spirit of a *cure,* a variety of therapies for treating the patient have been introduced (see Part II). Many, such as shock therapy, and lobotomies, were severe, in that they could damage the central nervous system. As long as the public believed that these procedures could lead to the solving of mental health problems, however, they were willing to allow the risks to be taken.

Unfortunately, during this period, many who were considered very *sick* (usually diagnosed as schizophrenic) went voluntarily or involuntarily to institutions for mental health help, but many did not respond well to the new techniques. The backlog of patients in the institutions began to mount, particularly in the state hospitals. Pessimism superseded optimism. By 1955 the mental health system had declined noticeably. That year the state hospitals reached their highest number of residents; there were 560,000 patients in state and country mental hospitals. Following is a study of one state hospital, which is typical of the process:

A State Hospital in the Process of Decline

In the 1930s and 40s this state hospital was considered one of the best agencies of its kind in the United States. It functioned out of a medical model; it had highly credentialed psychiatrists; it had a full psychiatric residency program; treatment was in the hands of specialists. It was indeed the golden age of the state hospital. Patients were carefully evaluated, specific treatment was developed, and within this system the staff attempted to deliver effective ser-

167

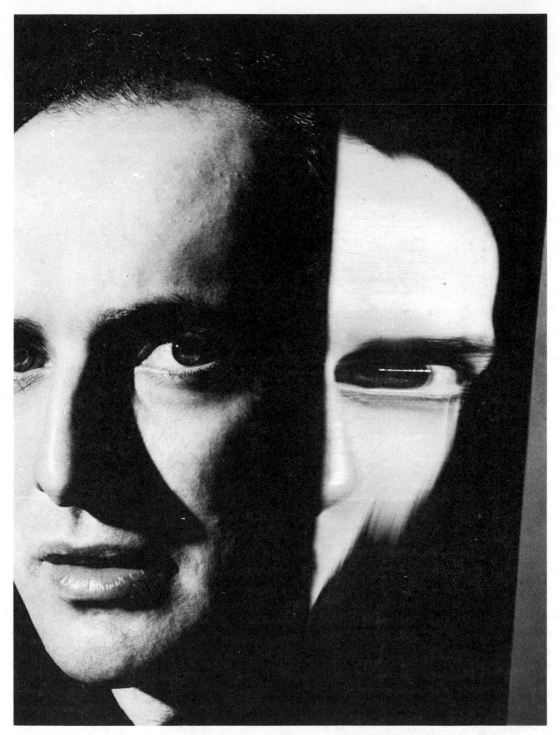

Optimism in the 1930s and 40s for "cures" turned to pessimism in the 1950s and 60s. (Photo by Bob Henriques, courtesy Magnum.)

vices. The hospital did not attempt to incorporate the psychoanalytical approach as its primary treatment and delivery system, but many of Sigmund Freud's concepts were important to the working of the system.

When a patient arrived at the hospital, there was never any question among the staff that here was a sick person. Patients were seen as victims of unconscious forces, hormonal imbalances, disturbed families, or neurological deficiencies. It was assumed that the patient could do little about his plight; he was merely a victim of his *illness*. He was to become the object of the action; he was to be *cured* by the expertise of the therapist.

During those years, the state hospital used the hospital-disease-cure approach. It attempted to diagnose each incoming patient. Initially it was more than simply placing labels; it was an effort to comprehend the inner operations of a person, to *tease out* the cause or causes of his malfunctioning, to prescribe treatment, discharge him, and, hopefully, follow up with aftercare.

Beginning of the Decline

The patient population was stable for a number of years. Most of the patients entering the hospital went through in a reasonable amount of time. Then the population began to increase, at first imperceptibly. Slowly but surely a group of patients who were described as poor prognostic risks—seriously impaired, homicidal, suicidal, with few resources—were pushed into the inner wards of the hospital where a residual population accumulated. Between 1930 and 1955 the hospital's inpatient population increased from 2,000 to nearly 7,000, while the staff of 900 increased only about one-third, with most of the increase occurring in the maintenance and custodial staff.

Under the circumstances, the hospital inevitably deteriorated, regardless of its good intentions. The initial attempt to diagnose and understand the nature of illnesses became perfunctory. It took two basic forms:

Each Monday morning a few staff physicians would go to the records office and quickly label each patient. There were certain wild-card labels—schizophrenic reaction, chronic undifferentiated type or personality pattern disturbance, inadequate personality.

A few, very few, patients identified as *classic*, or good prognostic risks, were elaborately evaluated. Each morning at least 75 percent of the professional staff gathered to evaluate one *classic* patient. These meetings lasted from 8:30 to about 10:30, with an informal discussion of the case often continuing until lunchtime. For a few patients, evaluation was excellent, but recommendations were followed through only infrequently.

As part of the deterioration, a tendency to isolate patients took hold of the hospital. This is a key theme in any service system and for that reason is worthy of explanation. Society has a strong tendency to banish, isolate, exile those who do not meet certain of its requirements: crimes lead to jail; deviance leads to mental hospitals; bad conduct leads to school expulsion. It would be silly to say there are no circumstances in which banishment and isolation are necessary. But if not carefully controlled isolation can become a means of eliminating basic responsibility. As the hospital under discussion became more and more crowded, the staff in the intake ward—following the example of private practitioners, general hospitals, community clinics, and school systems—expelled the less desirable patients and sent them deeper into the hospital system. As is true of most such systems, rising back up through the system is infinitely more difficult, particularly as the system becomes increasingly crowded.

The inner hospital wards became a custodial snake pit in spite of the treatment staff's best efforts. The continued application of traditional intraorganismic models of change, demanding large numbers of highly professional clinicians, led to the moral abandonment of many patients because they had been given a poor prognosis. The staff became somewhat desperate in their attempts to prevent patients from riding the assembly line to the back wards. Since most professional staff—the *therapists*—were placed in the reception wards in order to prevent patients from flowing to the inner hell, the back wards were practically abandoned and denied any possibility of being upgraded. Ward populations soared, there was little treatment of any kind, and the back ward care-takers became preoccupied with hygiene, orderliness and the avoidance of acting out through repressive measures. New patients were held in the reception wards as long as possible, which resulted in overcrowding, thus further reducing the effectiveness of treatment. Vicious circles, which drained staff effectiveness, were created throughout the hospital. In short, an uncontrolled chain reaction took place.

Approaching Collapse

As the hospital system deteriorated, hospital administrators became increasingly sensitive about the inner anarchy. Afraid of criticism, they left decision-making to the "super" experts. In this particular hospital, three men, all in administrative positions and infrequent visitors to the wards, made most of the formal decisions about the operation of the hospital and the fate of the patients. Even though these men had the best credentials, the superintendent felt he had to review all of their decisions. Assuming that they had an adequate amount of good judgement, they were simply overwhelmed by the enormity of their task. If any of them became ill or went on vacation, the already staggering system approached collapse. Important decisions were delayed or never made, and patients who might have been moved quickly through the system were held and more or less permanently institutionalized.

The backlog of patients convinced the staff that the patients were profoundly sick people. Treatment would have to be lengthy, careful, complex, and deep. Following this logic, the staff assumed that treatment could be undertaken only by elite therapists, of which the large public mental health facility had few. This situation led to the few therapists who *were* available involving themselves in complicated therapeutic relationships with a small number of patients, with most of the patients receiving little or no help.

The staff also assumed that these patients were no longer able to care for themselves, that they no longer had decision making abilities or could assume responsibility. Miniature authoritarian societies developed, which took over the responsibility and care of the patients. Since the staff were taking over responsibility for the lives of the patients, the hospital searched for specialists with impressive academic credentials who could make the crucial decisions. But at the same time, the salary and reputation of the hospital made it unattractive for the most qualified specialists.

In the late 1940s and early 50s the hospital reached its lowest point. It was unable to meet the standards of existing treatment

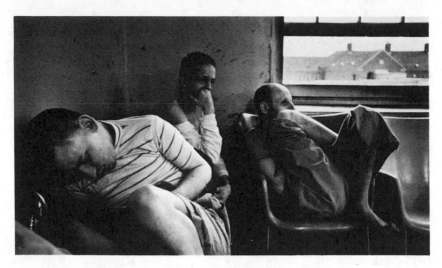

With the deterioration of the state hospitals, some patients were relegated to deeper parts of the hospital system. (Photo by Bill Stanton, courtesy Magnum.)

Imagine the frustrations of the disadvantaged person in some of today's hospitals. (Photo by Charles Harbutt, courtesy Magnum.)

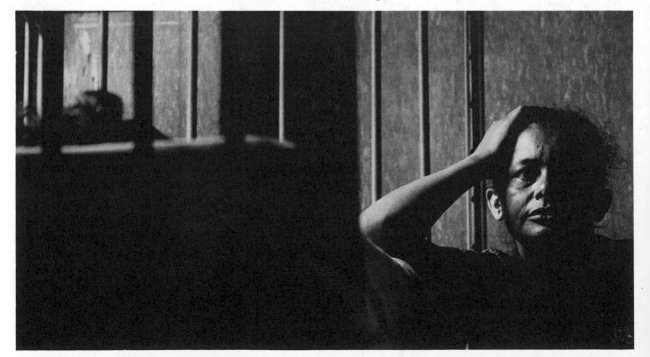

facilities such as general hospitals, private practitioners, and small, private, exclusive hospitals. Not being able to do this, the hospital lost its hospital accreditation; it lost its residency program; it saw its best staff dwindle away. Nevertheless, despite the deterioration for more than a decade, the hospital remained locked in its impotent posture, making few organized attempts to change.

What Went Wrong

As one examines the period 1930-55, it seems clear that during that time state hospitals served primarily disadvantaged persons. In the current idiom, these patients were *high-risk* patients. They had little education, little in the way of careers, poor ties to the economy, not much in the way of intimate relationships, and a poor social network. Under stress, they quickly demonstrated these char-acteristics—identity confusion, role confusion, and homicidal or suicidal patterns associated with psychoses. Most typically, when these patients entered the hospital for the first time, their behavioral patterns were classified as a form of acute schizophrenia. When they entered for the second or third time, they were labeled *chronic* schizophrenics. In sociological terms:

Disadvantaged persons have a limited number of options. They can maintain themselves at a marginal level indefinitely—accommodate themselves to the situation. They can attempt to link up with the mainstream of society via traditional procedures, for example, career ladders or the educational system. They can pursue a criminal career and attempt to use it as their career ladder. They can select deviance as a way of reacting to their everyday stress.

In the state hospital, the primary patients fall into the category mentioned last. Evidence of this is found in the works of August Hollingshead and Frederick Redlich [1965], as well as several un-published studies—Walter Fisher and Allen Laughlin [1964] and Walter Fisher and Joseph Mehr [1965].

These high-risk patients came to escape the stress patterns in their life–perhaps it was a cop-out. They took on the patterns of behavior that are a passport to a mental hospital. Norris Hansell [1970] refers to these external trappings as "frozen plumage."

The hospital received them into their "ports of entry"—variously called diagnostic centers, reception wards, and intake wards. These wards were most like general hospitals: physical examinations, laboratory work, diagnosis, prescriptions. In every sense, they were the best wards in the hospital—large staffs, good physical plant, active treatment programs, and hopeful attitudes.

In the context of the medical model staff attempted to examine the inner problems of the disadvantaged person. There was an attempt to find inner causes—neurological, chemical, psychological. If one was found, sophisticated intervention techniques were attempted to remove the cause of the illness.

Within this medical model hospital setting and within the structure of the disease model, the patient was forced to make a crossroads decision: recovery meant reasonably early discharge to his previous existence; acceptance of being a long-term patient meant descent into the snake pit and the eventual cutting of ties with his entire social network.

There was no attempt to examine the social situation and study its impact on the individual. Emphasis was on the initial attempt to treat the *disease.*

The increase in number of patients from 2,000 to 7,000 in 15 years was a prime indicator of failure of the system. It became clear that those patients who made a career of being patients were particularly vulnerable to the hospital-deterioration situation existing in such a massively bureaucratic institution. The patients declined in the institution—or perhaps in some ways, the institution declined along with the patients. The hospital set up a negative career ladder, which moved in only one direction. *Success* meant moving from the reception ward to the most regressed snake pit.

Although the professional staff gave the few intake wards their special flavor, the remainder of the hospital received its form and patterns primarily from the custodial staff and patients.

Reinforcement of Deviance

The patients found in those back ward ghettos a milieu to which they could adapt without much internal stress. The built-in reward-and-punishment system supported them in their adaptation. Crisis is the characteristic of growth (Erik H. Eriksen [1963]). Excitement, agitation, and disturbance are generally unacceptable on most hospital wards. That is, those behaviors most commonly associated with growth in the deviant individual are the least acceptable in the mental hospital. Behavioral patterns associated with chronicity, apathy, and hopelessness were the most acceptable; that is, those behaviors most associated with stagnation are the most acceptable in mental hospitals. Professional staff were called in only when the patient was unmanagable or in a crisis. The physician was called in to quiet the patient, which eliminated growth patterns (a quiet patient was a good patient).

Following are some items which express the built-in value system: (1) Since patients were not responsible for their behavior, they were not allowed to use forks and knives with their meals. Utensils were potentially dangerous weapons. This, of course, forced the patients to eat with their hands. It wasn't long before the staff began to describe the eating patterns of patients as being characteristic of their illness, as animal-like, which eventually became acceptable patient behavior. (2) Patient clothing rooms were set up with a monitor at the door to prevent theft. If a patient wanted to change his clothes, he had to get permission from the monitor to obtain his clothes. If the monitor was bothered too frequently, he gave the patients a hard time. Soon they stopped asking for a change of clothes, began to look dirty, and were described as being *messy*. Eventually the patients were *expected* to look that way. (3) All of those situations in the environment that required problem-solving and development of responsibility were removed from the patient's life. The patients were not allowed to handle their own money, participate in interpersonal relations with the opposite sex, move around in the environment on their own, or to participate in making decisions concerning their own destiny. They were no longer expected to be responsible.

Evaluation

The foregoing history of a state hospital is similar to the histories of most of the mental health agencies during that period. The model was not working, and it apparently wasn't working because of an expanding and changing target population. (We do not mean to

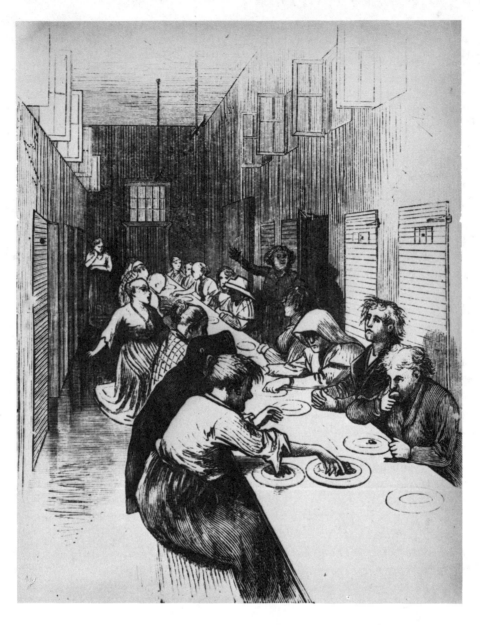

Insane poor at their meal in a state institution. Note the lack of eating utensils. (Courtesy the Bettmann Archives.)

imply that this traditional approach would not work for some patients.)

It was as if mental health workers were wearing blinders. They did not understand the nature of their task. They were attempting to mimic the functioning of the private, prestigous mental health facilities such as *Menninger's Clinic* and *Chesnut Lodge*, oblivious to the difference in resources and target populations. Prestige institutions provide staff ratios of five to one in direct-care staff; typically, a state hospital does not provide even one-to-one ratios. The medical model requires a high staff-to-patient ratio. Facilities such as Menninger's treat patients from the higher socioeconomic levels; state hospitals have always had the task of serving the high-risk patient, the disadvantaged, and the minorities. It is a different problem and requires different services. Failure to recognize the nature and scope of the task has contributed to the public mental health profession's lack of success in meeting the needs of their patients.

Summary

The medical model has been the dominant system for managing mental health deviance for the past 200 years. Out of it have come endless techniques and therapies, which, it was thought, could treat and cure behavior that is connected with mental illness.

There are no signs of an impending decrease in deviance. In fact, it appears that the problem is growing. The traditional systems are not working adequately. The target population is larger and more heterogenous than was previously thought. The most distressing aspect of this situation are the minimal attempts at evaluation and the few signs of effectiveness in systems that have been evaluated.

Chapter 12 Contributions to Decline and Failure

n Chapter 11 we described the decline of the mental health system within the medical-Freudian model. In this chapter we will discuss the factors that have contributed to this decline.

The Medical-Freudian Model

The assumptions of the medical-Freudian model led public mental health workers to the point where they were overwhelmed by the 1950s. Patient populations at institutions had soared and the dwindling staff were forced to abandon most of them. The concepts of the medical-Freudian model in contemporary society has brought the delivery systems to the point of collapse.

The Concept of Mental Illness

Not enough can be said about the issue of mental illness. As was stated earlier, it is an assumption of the medical-Freudian model that deviant behavior is caused by an inner disease. The problem is to locate the cause of the disease, prescribe appropriate treatment, and thus "cure" the patient. But this problem leads to others. It appears to be nearly impossible to identify one specific cause. Whether or not it is felt that the cause has been identified, in many instances the treatment has not been successful. It has become the conventional wisdom of mental health politics that those who do not respond to treatment are very *sick* (had a poor prognosis) and should be committed to mental hospitals. Once they are there, however, the process of institutionalization becomes the final process in maximizing deviance.

Target Population

In designing a treatment system, Freud was strongly influenced by his patients' style of life. The same is true of mental health experts today. Most mental health theories of the past 100 years were generated in private mental health centers, universities, and private practice. The patients in these institutions have typically been intelligent, high-resource, middle- and upper-class persons with well-developed personalities (energy, good appearance, goals).

For many years it has been assumed that these patients were the patients mental health workers are supposed to serve. Those patients who did not fit the pattern nor respond to the dominant methods of treatment disappointed mental health workers and were considered poor prognostic risks. Therapists considered it bad luck to be employed in an agency (such as a state hospital) that did not have *good* patients. Despite the fact that most of their patients were not the "right sort," state hospitals still maintained clinical programs designed for patients who had a good prognosis by standards of the medical-Freudian model. Those who did not respond to the model were shunted off to the back wards to live out their lives under snake-pit conditions while the state hospitals concentrated on those

179

The same poor socioeconomic conditions and societal breakdowns that drove these girls into their style of life are the background of many mental health patients today. (Photo by Burt Glinn, courtesy Magnum.)

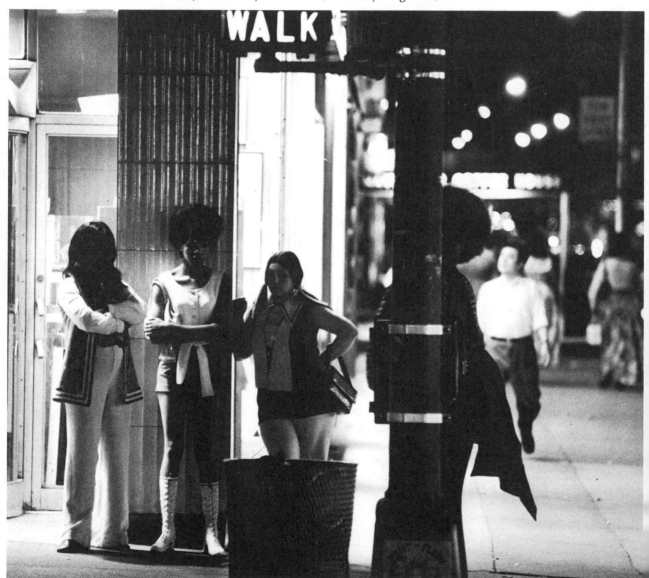

patients who had sufficient resources to make use of medical-Freudian treatment. This type of patient, however, represented a small minority of the population. As stated earlier, the state hospital had by the mid-50s become overcrowded with low-resource patients, which resulted in most of the services going to the patients with the least need, prestige agencies focusing on a minority mental health issue, and primary mental health issues being left to the institutions with the least prestige. It took many years to actually identify the target population. The typical mental health patient is female, aged 35 to 64, has less than a high school education, is separated or divorced, belongs to a family which earns $3,600 to $5,000 a year, and is in the low-middle to low socioeconomic class. This kind of patient requires services in order to survive.

All human service agencies—mental hospitals, schools, prisons, and welfare—now realize that their major target population is the unresponsive, involuntary, least competent persons, those who require more and different services than does the traditional target population.

The Inner Man

Adherents of the medical-Freudian approach assume that a person is maladaptive because of events which took place in that person's life. They further assume that if mental health workers are to aid (treat) patients, they must become expert about the *inner man*. At the heart of the issue is the process of detecting the inner factors that cause maladaptation, or deviancy. Although mental health workers thus far have misunderstood this inner psychological process, they continue to perform services as if they understood it perfectly. Neither have they been able to set operational goals; they are unable to get across to the patient what it is they are trying to do for him. Service-givers have condemned people who refuse the inner-search process or are unable to participate in it. They have ignored the impact of the immediate milieu on the individual. It is suggested that students read Kurt Lewin [1935] and B.F. Skinner [1938] in regard to understanding the influences of the individual's environment on his behavior.

A situation has developed in which therapists spend years examining the inner functioning of one person while hundreds, or possibly

181

thousands, go without services, and there is as yet no conclusive evidence that even these few inner searches are effective.

Techniques and Therapies

The medical-Freudian model concentrates on finding a special therapy for a disease. The usual answer to a problem is a *cure.* The recent history of the mental health field is almost like a pop culture; there are frequent reports of new therapies: gestalt, confrontation, psychodrama, transactional analysis, vitamin therapy, primal therapy, a new surgical procedure, a new convulsive therapy.

This technological concept of therapy had some value for the high resource people who had good jobs, families, friends, money, and good educational backgrounds. With these patients when you removed the symptom, they had a life style with which to relink. Libraries and book stores are filled with books on these techniques.

Unfortunately, such spectacular treatment is only a fraction of the services needed. Most patients not only have specific symptoms and problems, they have major life-style difficulties: poor education, poor job and interpersonal skills, few community resources, poor personality assets. Once you remove the symptoms, the task has only begun. The patient must be aided in developing the skills, abilities, and attitudes necessary to return to society and cope with life in it.

Failure to recognize the true therapeutic issues has resulted in a large number of patients lapsing into earlier deviant behavior, as is indicated in Table 12.1 from the National Institute of Mental Health, as well as much time being spent searching the inner man.

Table 12.1

Percent of Admissions with Previous Episodes of Care in Hospitals, State and County Mental Hospital Inpatient Services, United States, 1969

Age at admission	Percent with previous episode of care in the past 12 months.	Percent Over All Time
under 18	11.1	13.9
18-24	28.6	35.9
25-34	32.1	50.4
35-44	34.6	53.7
35-64	31.8	56.3
65 and over	10.4	30.1
all ages	28.2	47.1

Elitism: Supply and Demand

The medical-Freudian model requires expert therapists with impressive credentials. This is true not only of medical persons but also of psychologists, social workers, and nurses. In the past, it took a minimum of six years of university work to be able to provide therapy. To provide leadership for the therapeutic team, one must have approximately 15 years of education and training. Of course, the immediate result is a shortage of mental health workers. (Fin Arnhoff, E.A. Rubenstein, and J.C. Speisman [1969] believe that the shortage of professional workers is continuing to increase and that many professional positions are going unfilled.)

As long as adherence to elitism dominates the field, there will not be enough professionals to provide service. From 1950 to 1966, the number of professionals increased—psychiatrists 350 percent, psychologists 500 percent, social workers 400 percent, and psychiatric nurses 250 percent (Arnhoff, Rubenstein, Shriver, and Jones [1969]). Despite these increases, a shortage of highly credentialed staff continues. It was and is the pattern in mental health to omit therapeutic services when there is an insufficient number of persons with credentials. If patients, the public, and service-givers continue to favor elitism, there will be an increasing imbalance between service-givers and those who need mental health services.

Evaluation

Various mental health groups have grown impatient with the lack of therapists while at the same time, there is no hard evidence that the treatment programs are effective. It is ironic that one should develop elite, expensive therapy while at the same time not provide evidence of the effectiveness of the service.

For a long time, it has been hinted that with sufficient money, training, and staff, it would be possible to cure deviance and improve community mental health. But mental health has been committed to a utopian dream. It is this theme that has perhaps been the most important factor in setting the stage for the decline of traditional mental health services.

Other Factors

There are many themes in the medical-Freudian model that have contributed to the crisis in the mental health system, but other cultural forces have also contributed to the crisis. The third revolution in mental health has been affected by politics, sociology, and economics, as well.

The Momentum of Change

Change in society accelerates with the accumulation of knowledge. Western society has changed more in the past century than in the entire history of mankind. Values and beliefs that appeared so firm in the 1920s and 30s have become the cliches of the 1970s. Once cherished institutions such as church, family, and marriage appear to be becoming obsolete. There no longer appears to be stable attitudes toward sex, violence, love, and hate. Most adults in their thirties and above probably suffer from value or cultural shock. The great culture taboos against incest, patricide, cannibalism, matricide, and homosexuality, which Freud saw as the basic themes repressed by man, can now be seen in one's local movie theater. Not only are we going through a rapid process of change, but the process itself is gathering momentum. Most theories and models in this century are being questioned and challenged. A rapidly changing society requires new approaches to explain and predict human behavior.

The Process of Change

Although most people sense the changes going on around them, they know little about the forces that cause the changes and govern their course. Historically, society has given names to the manifestations of change—the Renaissance, the revolution of rising expectations, the third revolution in mental health. Individuals in a society appear helpless to affect the process of social change. This is true for those who want to speed up change as well as those who prefer to maintain the status quo. Even now, as we view the mental health model, it is impossible to predict its thrust or direction in the future.

The reader can probably best understand this from a historical perspective. The Freudian model began near the end of the 19th century, in a period characterized by Puritanical and repressive child-rearing. Freud's therapy model focused on reducing inhibitions and returning the repressed to consciousness, an approach that was angrily resisted. An examination of Freud's later works [1950] and the historical text of Ernest Jones [1957] indicate that the social resistance and anger had a major negative impact on the acceptance of Freud's ideas.

But in retrospect, it seems clear that Freud was in the forefront of major societal changes in values, attitudes, and philosophies. Society was changing, and the existing child-rearing practices and human service practices were no longer appropriate. It was time for a change. The authors suggest that today it is again time for a change and that current mental health delivery models and techniques are insufficient to meet today's mental health needs. Following are some of the developing attitudes and their implication for existing mental health approaches:

Because of Nazi intolerance and policies of genocide, it became less popular to discriminate against minorities and the disadvantaged. Racial minorities, women, the mentally ill, and the poor were to receive something closer to their fair share of social services than they had before. It was no longer fashionable to lock up atypical persons in mental hospitals and forget about them.

The minority and disadvantaged young men who had fought for their country were no longer willing to live in their prewar ghettos. They had had an opportunity to see the world, and they now wanted more out of life than their parents had had. They wanted the same services the middle and upper classes received. Separate hospitals and clinics for the poor were no longer acceptable. It had become clear that as long as mental health services were different for the poor, the poor were going to receive inferior services. Many young people who had never received health services became acquainted

185

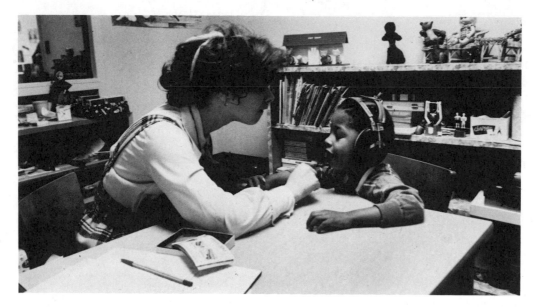

Human services agencies have realized that their major
target population is no longer the elite, but the
underprivileged, unresponsive groups of society.
(Courtesy Lexington School for the Deaf.)

The "typical" mental health patient today is female,
aged 35-64, has less than a high school education, is
separated or divorced, and belongs to a family that
earns $3,600 to $5,000 a year. (Photo by Charles Harbutt,
courtesy Magnum).

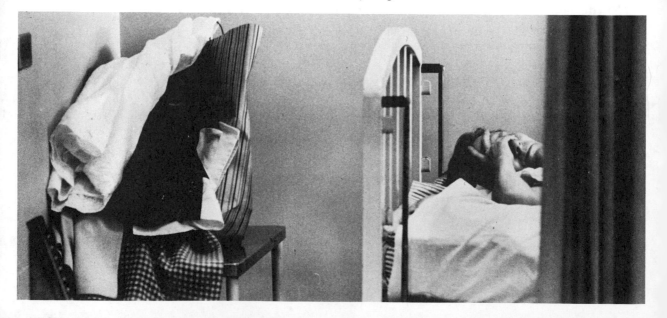

with the possibilities while they were in the armed forces. It became part of their lives, and they felt that they and their families deserved such help. Health services were no longer considered a privilege; they were a right. Suddenly many more were seeking the service than there were services available—a classic situation which demanded change. If we were going to deliver the elite service to everyone, health services would inevitably be in a crisis.

There was a great demand for participation. Soldiers returning from the war wanted to have a say in the decision-making of their society. As part of having been in the army, they now felt a sense of activism. *If you don't like the way things are, change them.* (For those who want to experience this feeling, we suggest they see the movie, *The Best Years of our Lives.*) This postwar spirit was very much at odds with the mental health models of those days. The mental health professions took the position that doctor knows best; if someone is not behaving adequately, it means he is sick and must be cured. But the new spirit suggested that it was not the individual who was sick, it was society.

A new breed of social scientists appeared. Instead of examining deviance and behavioral disorders as being those solely of the individual, they began to focus on society. All of society's systems were opened to evaluation and criticism: prisons, schools, health care, mental hospitals. E. Goffman [1961], in a muckraking fashion, describes the impact of institutionalization by detailing its destructive force on the individual. Martin [1955] and Wing [1962] suggest that many of the characteristics we ascribe to psychiatric illness are actually caused by existing systems in mental hospitals—stripping of personal identity, removal of decision-making, stripping of responsibility, disengagement from the social network, separation from the cash economy, and being pushed into a strange world with a minimal structure. The institutionalized person who has been robbed of his past has little alternative but to take on the new identity of Patienthood.

Obsolete Techniques

The therapeutic techniques that had been developed for the middle and upper classes were useless for meeting the needs of the new patients. The disadvantaged did not want to spend time investigating their inner selves; it was no longer a fashionable or reasonable

187

thing to do. They wanted help as well as therapy. It appeared that if service workers were to help the disadvantaged person, they would have to do it by altering his environment and not just his inner self. It was a time for new service models.

New Social Movements

In the 1950s and 60s American society saw the development of important new social movements: civil rights, consumerism, and women's liberation, to name a few. Each has brought about changes in society that have benefited members of various previously scapegoated and disadvantaged groups. Each has provided an activist orientation, in contrast to the passivity of traditional mental health models. The disadvantaged have demanded more aggressive action and quicker changes. It is quite likely that these new social movements have provided more services to maladaptive persons than have the mental health models.

The Revolution of Rising Expectations

Society has learned in the past 25 years that when you help the oppressed to improve their lot, this does not reduce their expectations; it raises them. When you elevate the disadvantaged in the social structure, it intensifies their demands for improvement and equalization.

Summary

In this chapter we have attempted to identify the social forces gathering to make the traditional medical model obsolete. The services being offered are incongruent with the needs of society. It is crucial to all systems to be able to identify and meet the needs of the patient.

Pandora's box has been opened in American society. Everyone wants more of the action and a greater portion of the pie. This country is being plunged into crisis by the "tide of rising expectations." The disadvantaged and the minorities are no longer willing to sit back and accept a status quo which disenfranchises and alienates them. The rising expectations permeate every phase of life, every social institution. The service agencies, the universities, and most service systems have not yet begun to make the alterations in their models necessary to accommodate these new attitudes and expectations.

Chapter 13 Outgrowths of Failure

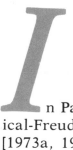n Part III we have been focusing on the decline of the medical-Freudian model. W. Fisher, J. Mehr, and P. Truckenbrod [1973a, 1973b,] have described this decline as a *critical mass* situation. The concept of critical mass is an interesting analogy of the failure of most human service agencies in the past 20 years.

Critical Mass

In the two papers by Fisher, Mehr, and Truckenbrod, they describe critical mass:

The concept, Critical Mass, refers to a general notion in nuclear engineering which has relevance . . . to our own field of mental health. It concerns the minimum amount of radioactive material needed to sustain a chain reaction. All radioactive material decomposes because of an inherent instability . . . of the nucleus. The decomposition (or emission) of neutrons . . . is what makes a particular element or isotope radioactive. Under normal conditions, decomposition is at an orderly, extremely precise rate. When enough radioactive material gets together, the neutrons from the decomposing atoms . . . strike the nucleus of other atoms (causing them to decompose) and a chain reaction is set in motion. Of the two types of chain reactions, controlled reactions are used for the purpose of generating energy in the form of heat, while in any uncontrolled nuclear chain reaction, the process is rapid and creates huge amounts of energy in a very short time. This, of course, is how an atomic bomb operates.

There seems to be a basic analogy to this nuclear engineering concept in mental health delivery systems in general. Static systems (those unresponsive to basic needs) which continue to utilize traditional responses to pressing demands, quickly become overloaded by their input processes, eventually reaching a chain-reaction level.

The critical mass situations in large urban centers are related to the absolute number of consumers—patients, students, and the disadvantaged—seeking services. Just as critical mass in nuclear engineering is dependent on a variety of factors, however, so is critical mass in the social sciences linked to a number of variables. The following quote from W.E. Moore [1963], while not written with critical mass in mind, articulates portions of the concept very well:

Yet if the contemporary world is not uniformly chaotic, there are complexities in social change that are likely to manifest themselves as *tensions* and *strains*. Persistent patterns in one field of action may eventually collide with trends in another—for example, the persistent pattern that impels nearly everyone to go to work at the same hour in the morning may be increasingly inconsistent with the urban growth, the resulting strains being reflected in overloaded transportation facilities and traffic congestion.

Although one cannot accurately quantify critical mass situations in the social sciences and the human services, decomposition and subsequent instabilities develop in social systems which cannot meet the needs of the public they are supposed to serve. Mental health facilities do not evolve entirely through systematic or deliberate design. Agencies such as the state hospital described in Chapter 12 are shaped by historical custom, with its rigidities, trial-and-error adaptations, and many subtle pressures.

191

How the Public Influences Agencies

- Citizens apply various pressures because they want to: get dangerous noncriminals off the streets and keep them off; get their relatives home as quickly as possible; spend as little money as possible; find new, creative treatment; let anyone who applies enter the hospital.
- State governors, as part of the public, have prodded agencies in many directions.
- Legislators, also as part of the public, have from time to time applied shifting pressures.
- Patients have not responded to available therapeutic techniques.
- State hospitals also have a less influential constituency applying pressures: research workers, universities, mental health professionals, unions, treatment theorists, other mental health facilities, local communities, and the courts.
- As long as trial-and-error adaptation meets the pressures, an agency remains stable. When a mental health system does not meet its basic pressures adequately, however, a *symptom pattern* (the critical mass situation), develops.

Decline and Breakdown

- The staff develops pessimism, apathy, and a sense of despair.
- The quality of the staff, measured by the standards of the particular period, decline.
- The residential and/or nonresidential population significantly increases, reaching a point where treatment is no longer possible.
- Staff to-patient ratios decline.
- The greatest turnover in personnel occurs among the more skilled staff.
- The primary service goals of the agencies are minimized, and the professional staff focuses on secondary functions such as training.
- The agency receives a smaller share of the budget, and physical plant and equipment deteriorate.
- The remaining staff are not competent to use the existing therapies.
- The number of treatment programs declines, and the care-givers become increasingly involved in maintenance and custodial duties.

• There is a growing tendency to isolate patients. Unable to manage patients, the community quickly exiles them to residential facilities. Programs within the facility, unable to manage them either, force them to the more regressed wards.

• The continuity of treatment disappears; patients are transferred, the staff transfers, yet there are no attempts to develop appropriate communication and therapeutic links between the previous caregivers and the new ones.

As we stated, critical mass has become apparent in the human service fields in the past two decades. In the remainder of this chapter, newspaper headlines, with brief comments, will be used to focus attention on the failures.

ECCENTRIC OR INSANE? MENTAL HEALTH COURT ANGUISH. This headline reflects the current anguish and confusion of the courts in determining who should be committed to mental institutions. Fifteen or twenty years ago it was taken for granted that those who behaved atypically or maladaptively were *sick*. It was obvious that a physician, a person trained in the pathology of illness, could most appropriately make commitment decisions. Throughout most of this century physicians' recommendations in such matters have rarely been questioned.

The human service revolution has provided a new perspective. It can no longer be taken for granted that all who have delusions or hallucinations belong in mental institutions. Mental health workers have become increasingly concerned about patients' civil rights, as well as their right to treatment. Why keep them in a mental hospital if they are not dangerous to themselves or to others? Why keep them there if the hospital cannot provide treatment or if they are unable to respond to the services mental health workers can provide?

More than any other mental health worker, Thomas Szasz [1961, 1971], is responsible for the reconsideration of the status and role of the mental health patient. We quote from an earlier book of ours (Fisher, Mehr, and Truckenbrod [1973c]):

Szasz feels that patients, like other minorities, e.g., women, children, and blacks, are scapegoated out of a societal paternalism. In effect, mental health workers are constantly locking up, exiling, and overtreating, supposedly for the sake of the individual and the greater society. Szasz suggests

193

Violent manifestations of the strains and tensions of
urban living brought about by the deterioration of social
systems. (Below, photo by Leonard Freed, courtesy
Magnum; opposite, photo by Charles Harbutt, courtesy
Magnum.)

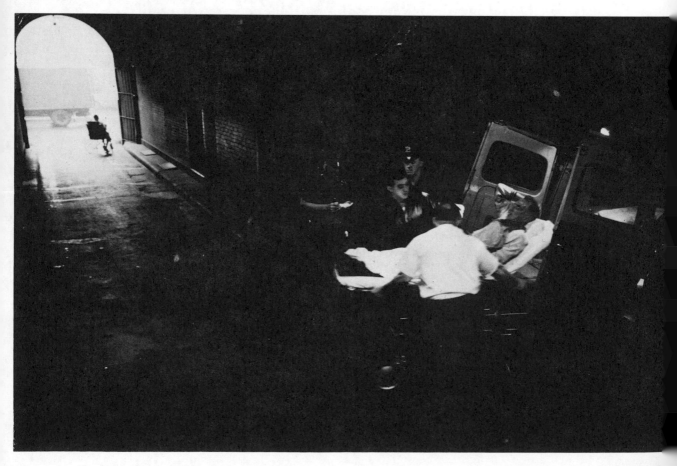

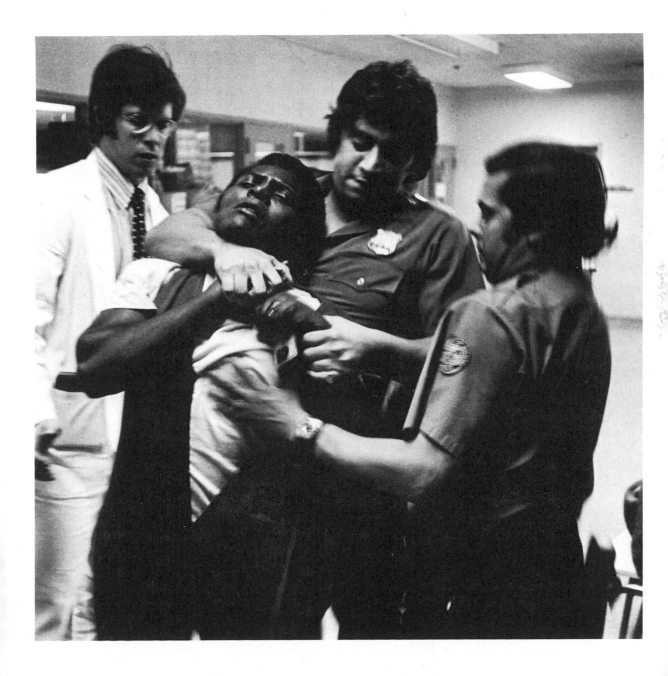

that out of our need to protect mental patients, society has given caregivers extra legal powers, which has . . . resulted in the violation of the involuntary patient's rights. Some of the implications [of Szasz's position] are evident in the following points:

1. There is no such thing as mental illness in the sense that one should *assume* that strange behavior results from a "disease process."

2. The individual can make any decision pertaining to himself so long as it does not hurt other people.

3. People who violate the law should go to a correctional institution and not a mental hospital.

4. Suicide is a personal decision.

5. Psychoanalysis is a form of religion.

6. Involuntary patients are a persecuted minority.

7. Declaring persons incompetent or mentally ill is an expression of a power struggle.

It seems fair to say that there is no definition of mental illness which effectively or operationally clarifies who should be in a mental hospital, who should be in prison, who should be in treatment, or who is normal. We typically end up with definitions under which everyone is mentally ill or no one is mentally ill.

In the summer of 1972 the ultimate confusion about mental illness became apparent in the furor over Senator Thomas Eagleton, the short-lived vice-presidential candidate of the Democratic Party. Shortly after his selection it became known that he had once been treated for *psychiatric problems*. He had, in fact, received electric shock treatment. Numerous questions arose. Had he been mentally ill? Was he still ill? Did his previous condition make it unlikely that he could function effectively if he should ever become President? If you once had emotional problems, would you always have emotional problems? Are those who seek mental health help *sicker* than those who do not?

No one can unequivocally answer these questions. In the past, those working from elitist models (such as the medical-Freudian) have acted as if they believed such questions could be answered expertly and precisely. But the inability to respond intelligently and appropriately to such questions has contributed to the loss of public trust and a reaction against the medical-Freudian model. It would seem that the traditional procedures for dealing with these problems are no longer effective.

These following newspaper comments on the problem of distinguishing between *mentally ill* and *mentally healthy* provide further insight into the problem.

CAN HOSPITALS REALLY TELL WHO'S INSANE? In an article under this headline (which appeared in a Stanford, California newspaper) Professor David L. Rosenhan, a Stanford University psychologist, said that he and seven other sane investigators (psychiatrist, pediatrician, painter, housewife, psychology graduate student, 3 psychologists) had arranged, as a test, to be admitted as schizophrenic patients in 12 different mental hospitals around the country. These hospitals were in California, Oregon, Pennsylvania, New York, and Delaware. *None of the eight was found to be sane by hospital professionals.* But, Rosenhan said, it was "quite common" for actual psychiatric patients to correctly identify the imposters. Rosenhan and his seven colleagues were eventually released as "schizophrenics in remission" despite their best efforts to convince the hospital staff of their sanity. "We now know that we cannot distinguish insanity from sanity," Rosehan said. "We continue to label patients 'schizophrenic,' 'manic depressive,' and 'insane' as if in those words we had captured the essence of understanding. We have known for a long time that our diagnoses often are not useful or reliable, but we have nevertheless continued to use them." Rosenhan said that the hospital itself imposes a special environment in which the meaning of behavior can easily be misunderstood. "The uniform failure to recognize sanity cannot be attributed to the quality of treatment facilities. While there was considerable variability between them, several are considered excellent. Nor can it be alleged that there simply was not enough time to observe the pseudopatients. Length of hospitalization ranged from seven to 52 days, with an average of 19 days. All pseudopatients took extensive notes publicly. Under ordinary circumstances such behavior would have raised questions in the minds of observers, as in fact it did among patients. Nursing records for three pseudopatients indicate that the writing was seen as an aspect of their pathological behavior."

Following are excerpts from an article which appeared in many newspapers:

DOCTORS FOR DEFENSE CALL BREMER INSANE. Arthur H. Bremer decided last March [1972] to assassinate either President Nixon or Alabama Gov. George C. Wallace, a pyschiatrist testified.

The defense psychiatrist described Bremer as a dispassionate schizophrenic, both methodical and careless and as being rejected by a teenage girl.

"He fantasized that when he fired his gun at President Nixon or Gov. Wallace, he would cry out, 'A penny for your thoughts.'"

The psychiatrist said he considered the 21-year-old defendant legally insane when, as prosecution eyewitnesses said, he wounded Wallace and three other persons with a pistol . . . at a Laurel, Maryland shopping center.

A second defense psychiatrist said she considered Bremer . . . a legally insane, latent schizophrenic affected by a "very serious blurring of the bounds between fantasy and reality."

"I believe he should be committed to a mental hospital to protect himself from his suicidal tendencies and to protect society from his homicidal tendencies," she testified.

The opinion of the two psychiatrists was in direct conflict with prosecution psychiatrists, who said that while Bremer had a mental disorder and was mixed up, he could, as Maryland insanity law requires, appreciate the criminality of his conduct and could conform to the law.

While the defense psychiatrist maintained that the former busboy and school janitor was a schizophrenic, the prosecution doctors said Bremer had the less severe disorder known as schizoid personality.

Bremer had pleaded innocent by reason of insanity to a 17-count indictment arising from the shootings. Under cross-examination, the defense psychiatrist said Bremer did not admit firing the gun at the shopping center at Laurel. "He told me about having the gun in his hand. He did not say he shot it."

The second defense psychiatrist said she had difficulty believing Bremer's admission to her that he shot Wallace and took the defendant's statements "with a big spoonful of salt."

She testified Bremer strove to become important to gain his mother's love and that "his idea to kill the President . . . was to impress her and have her look up to him."

The first defense psychiatrist said he had isolated distinct emotional crises in Bremer's life, the first at age 9, when against his wishes, his family moved on short notice. The second came about nine years later when Bremer, heretofore submissive at home, began challenging his parents, complaining about food and conditions, and finally moving away, according to the doctor. The third event, the "main crisis" in Bremer's life: rejection last winter by a 16-year-old girl, described . . . earlier . . . as the first and only person to whom Bremer had tried to relate closely. The rejection first led to a plan to commit mass murders and suicide and, when this was not carried out, to a mind-purging decision. "His rejection by his girl friend was terminated by his decision to assassinate the President."

We have included this article in order to make several points: (1) the psychiatrists' testimony conflicted; (2) the psychiatric testimony reflected the needs of those who employed the psychiatrists; (3) the psychiatric opinion, in that the individual experts interpreted the results differently, was generally subjective. It appears obvious that the question of sanity and insanity cannot be interpreted on an objective, operational, scientific basis.

American society today is riddled with violence. In a sense, a critical mass situation is rapidly developing. Anyone alive in the second half of the 20th century does not need to be reminded that hostility is rampant. When people cannot safely walk the streets at night, it is clear that there is a critical mass situation of rage and hostility. The attempt to reduce social rage by treating violent people one by one is like trying to make fresh water out of the Pacific Ocean drop by drop.

Desperate because the medical-Freudian orientation apparently has not reduced the violence in our society, experts have come up with new plans for stronger censorship, longer prison terms, and the return to capital punishment. The following newspaper reports indicate this trend: CASTRATE RAPISTS AND REVIVE DEATH PENALTY: BILLY GRAHAM; NIXON ASKS DEATH PENALTY, RESTRICTED INSANITY DEFENSE; PRESIDENT SENDS A 680-PAGE CRIMINAL CODE TO CONGRESS.

In the light of the fact that mental health agencies have not been able to demonstrate an appreciable effect on these problems, it is not surprising that alternatives to mental health solutions are being offered.

Violence is only one of our massive human service problems. Not long ago, Governor Nelson Rockefeller of New York said, "we must declare war on drugs." In effect, Rockefeller was saying that society must employ warlike tactics in this struggle. He wants the judicial system to give drug pushers long prison sentences with little chance for parole. He was not suggesting a mental health approach; instead, he was recommending that the problem is one for the police and correctional institutions.

Another newspaper article: "The United Auto Workers and Chrysler Corp. announced the establishment of a full-time narcotics treatment and rehabilitation program at the Chrysler gear and axle plant in Detroit." This speaks for itself. The drug problem appears to be of such severity that employers and unions have had to move into the human service field.

Our society appears to be overrun by deviance, crime, poverty, pollution, violence, and addiction. All systems are malfunctioning.

Yet despite the endless critical mass problems, traditional service-givers in almost all areas of human service insist on maintaining the status quo. This does not mean, for example, that education, mental health, and correctional institutions are not changing; rather it is that there are no *meaningful* changes. Most mental health systems continue to function in the manner described in Part II.

If the medical-Freudian orientation is proving inadequate, what are the alternatives? For one thing, society can move toward stronger security patterns—increase repression, build more jails, hire more guards, impose more severe sentences, restrict freedoms. There are strong trends in this direction. Historically most societies have used severe punitive measures without success. The failure of capital punishment to deter murder is the classic example of the ineffectiveness of the punishment-and-repression model.

In Part IV we will present the human service model (the third revolution in mental health) as an alternative to the medical-Freudian orientation. The following quote from Senator Walter F. Mondale [1972] is relevant to this theme:

Human services are becoming so central to the basic fabric of our society that their development is crucial in the transition from an industrial-wage society to a service-support society. That transition is required by the rapid transformation of our industry to automation, by our expanding population, and by the needs of individuals to be employed in ways that increasingly must yield satisfaction other than salary.

Thus my prediction is that an unprecedented expansion of the human services will characterize the 1970's. This expansion will cut across the fields of health, recreation, corrections, and employment. It will reach out to all age groups, on to urban and non-urban America alike. It will be erratic, to be sure, but [it] will be supported by all of the body politic.

This is not to say that the millenium has yet arrived, or that our glaring internal problems are on the verge of solution. It is to say that the human services must be viewed as a complex system, filling the needs of a society in which surplus labor abounds (as fewer people with increasingly specialized training are needed), which thereby requires more focused leisure, but which continues to support the work ethic as a central premise.

It is still true that one is identified by his or her occupation, that most people want to be gainfully employed, and that those deprived of work—for example, through early retirement—suffer psychological and physical disabilities. In short, one's worth is dependent upon one's work. So it is that at least one-half of our society, the female half, is engaged in a movement to equalize work, and, as a consequence, self worth. So, too, is it that social, psychological, political, and economic forces will lead to increasing utilization of the human services to fill the needs of a changing society. The human services industry, then, will have to bring health and social services to unserved populations, to manage the rebuilding of the cities, and to redevelop those regions of the country that are dying.

It is reasonable to predict that five million new community service jobs will be created in the next years. Jobs will be developed within occupational categories drawn from the new career efforts of the anti-poverty, health, and model cities programs. Hopefully, all will be related to career development ladders, connected closely with situations of higher education, and will build a living bridge between the needs of communities and the service activities of college and universities.

Senator Mondale's words express the main thrust of this book. The medical-Freudian orientation is not an effective solution to the critical mass situation. It is too expensive, too complex, and too demanding of the patient. Yet the punitive response to man's rising hopes ignores the vitality and progress of the changing social system. In Part IV the focus will be on the human service orientation.

Summary

The service systems have for some time been moving toward a state of disorganization and confusion. We call this confusion and disorganization a *critical mass* situation. It isn't only that service agencies have more problems but that the conflict over the appropriate services has intensified. Most service agencies find themselves caught between opposing forces. On one hand, there are strong civil rights groups who are pushing for greater freedom and permissiveness; on the other are many security-conscious groups who feel controls must be imposed by police-like action.

Even as this struggle continues, the critical mass situation expands. The crime rate continues to rise. State hospitals have sharply reduced their daily inpatient population while the number of acute disturbances rises. More people are seeking mental health services than ever before. The degree of cynicism and disenchantment in the United States continues to rise. In the context of these service-system crises, a new enterprise, the human service system, is emerging as a possible solution to the problem.

Part IV

The Human Service Model

Chapter 14 *The Development of the Human Service Model in a Troubled Culture*

The human service model is a pragmatic one—if something works, use it. The model is oriented toward problem-solving, with an emphasis on the here-and-now problems of the troubled person and the human service worker's willingness to try to cope with all facets of the person and his problems. It provides a new direction in thinking about what can be done in providing efficient mental health service to the emotional-social casualty. As was pointed out, this approach emerged because of the inadequacies in many areas of the traditional service systems. The following case history is an example of these inadequacies.

The Forgotten Man

This sad and true story begins in late 1953. A young black man, whom we will call George, heard from his family that his mother was ill. George was concerned about his mother and wanted to go home to see her, which was a thousand miles away. But he had little money. He started out hitchhiking. His first ride took him to an all-white, well-to-do suburb about 6:30 in the morning. George was large, extremely muscular, and very black. Within a few minutes he was spotted by the local police and after a brief struggle was put in jail.

As the days went by, George became more and more worried about his mother, in addition to the lack of action about his imprisonment. After a week, he lost patience and attacked one of the guards who tried to keep him from escaping. After he was subdued and restrained, a local physician decided that he was psychotic and needed to be hospitalized. He was transferred to an intake ward of the nearby state hospital where he was placed on the "assembly line": x-rays, urine analysis, physical examination, psychiatric examination, and diagnosis. A prognosis was made. At this point, in effect, his name was changed from George to "Schizophrenic." The usual treatment was prescribed: hydrotherapy, packs, chemotherapy, electric shock. But again, George couldn't tolerate imprisonment. He smashed the ward door down, picked up a steel pipe, and headed toward a nearby river, with the hospital security guard and the state police in pursuit. As George approached the river, a state policeman shot him in the leg.

It became the consensus of the staff that George was a dangerously sick man, and he was transferred to a security hospital of the state department of mental health. Soon everyone forgot George. The incident became merely another of a long series of such incidents in the hospital system. Most who knew of him assumed that George was eventually treated and released from the hospital. Ten years later, though, he was returned from the hospital to the state hospital as a manageable patient. The *treatment* had "taken." George was a true *Schizophrenic*—passive, manneristic, totally dependent on the institution, and frightened. He had become a full-fledged citizen of the state hospital. Since then, George has left the hospital many times to go to sheltered-care facilities, only to have to return to the state hospital after short periods of freedom. This pattern has become his life: going and coming, chemotherapy, chastisement for his failures, behavioral patterns classified as psychotic.

From the beginning, George's problems were human service ones. He was out of money. He had no communication with his

205

family. He was made a scapegoat by society because he had no money or friends and because he was black. There was no one to help him. Once he was labeled *sick*, George was placed on the mental health treadmill, which he had been riding for 20 years.

In many ways George's story reflects the circumstances surrounding the "third revolution in mental health," which has set the stage for a human services system.

A National Mental Health Program

By the late 1950s it was becoming clear that initiative and planning in mental health care must take place at a national level. This initiative was set forth in President Kennedy's message to Congress on February 5, 1963:

I propose a national mental health program to assist in the inauguration of a wholly new emphasis and approach to care for the mentally ill. This approach relies primarily upon the new knowledge and the new drugs acquired and developed in recent years which make it possible for most of the mentally ill to be successfully and quickly treated in their communities and returned to a useful place in society.

These breakthroughs have rendered obsolete the traditional methods of treatment which imposed upon the mentally ill a social quarantine, a prolonged or permanent confinement in huge, unhappy mental hospitals where they are out of sight and forgotten . . . We need a new type of health facility, one which will return mental health care to the mainstream . . . and at the same time upgrade mental health services.

This message, and the Community Mental Health Act of 1963 which followed, established a new set of priorities and social policies for the mentally ill and mentally retarded. President Kennedy's message and the legislation supporting it reaffirmed that all citizens are entitled to effective mental health treatment, which would be on a par with physical health care and should be provided in the citizen's own community. This new emphasis on community-based mental health services has made it necessary to change the existing large state hospitals and construct new community mental health centers where none existed before. The new focus on a community-based care model has also led to growing realization that the public has a responsibility for mental health services in their community, from both a financial and a decision-making standpoint.

At this point, it will be useful to take a more detailed look at how two different mental health systems recruited and deployed their available manpower in an effort to deal with the mandate in President Kennedy's message to Congress. We will present two brief histories of mental health agencies, which will give you an overview of the new orientation toward mental health and mental illness. Both agencies were moving toward a human service model. The first of these agencies was a new mental health zone center which was organized in a community with few existing mental health services. The second was a large state mental hospital which was transformed from a primarily custodial institution to a programmatic, service-oriented agency. Both agencies have worked toward providing effective mental health care, but started at quite different points. As you will see, one of them, primarily because of its newness, had a relatively unlimited budget for developing its staff. This is unusual; it is not typical of what other mental health agencies have to work with. The *economy*, in terms of funds for personnel, are typically never enough and nearly always represent a genuine poverty situation, which was the case with the second agency, the state hospital. Interestingly, both agencies encountered problems in their attempt to move the focus of treatment from that of a medical to a human services model. These problems stemmed largely from the expectations of the care-givers themselves about what good treatment should be, as well as from the training they had received in college and graduate school.

The Mental Health Zone Center

The mental health zone center was organized in the mid-1960s in a metropolitan area where there had been little federal- or state-supported mental health services. The center started out with the best of intentions to provide effective mental health services to the citizens of the community for which it was responsible. Staff were hired, and the typical agency bureaucracy was developed, complete with director, executive committee, clinical advisory committee,

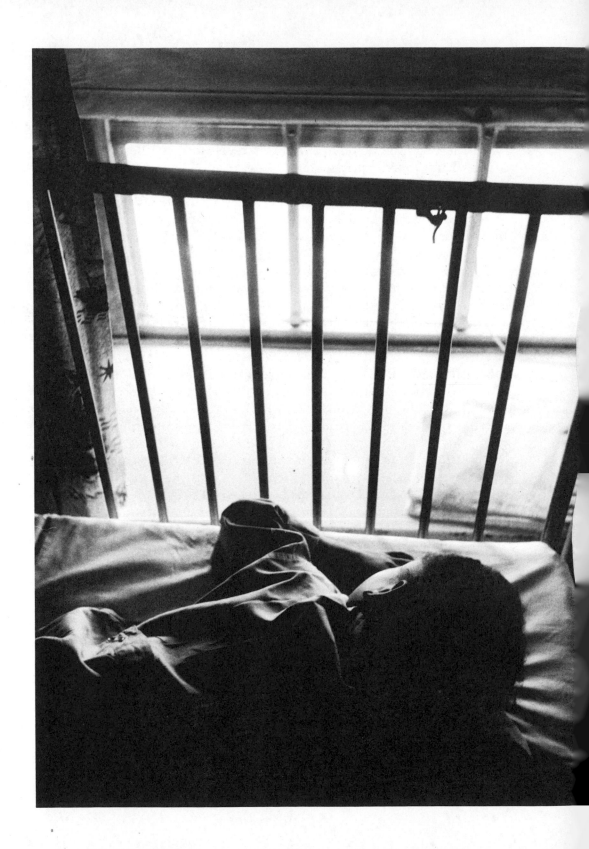

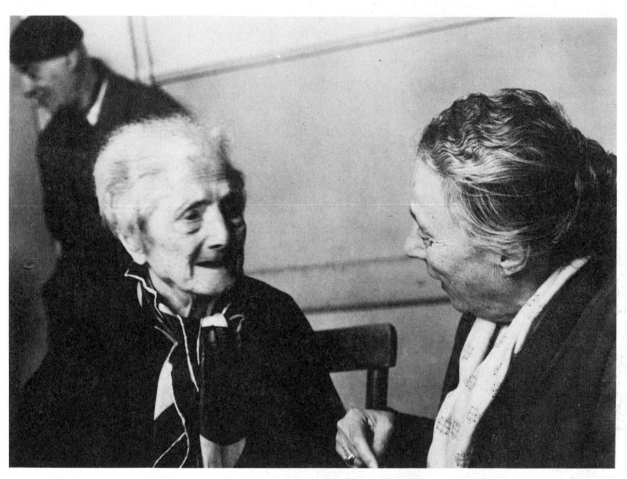

The aged are frequently handicapped by psychological stress as well as socioeconomic disruption. Refugees have unique problems which require understanding and warmth. (Photo from a Jewish home for transmigrants in Rome, Italy. Courtesy United Jewish Appeal.)

" . . . Breakthroughs have rendered obsolete the traditional methods of treatment which imposed on the mentally ill a social quarantine, a prolonged or permanent confinement in huge, unhappy mental hospitals where they are out of sight and forgotten . . . ." From President John F. Kennedy's message to Congress, February 5th, 1963. (Photo by Charles Harbutt, courtesy Magnum.)

clinical program directors, and, of course, the clinical staff members themselves. There was a professionalism evident, with each profession and service jealously guarding its territory.

A residential crisis intervention service opened with 30 beds and traveling teams which were supposed to go out into the community to provide aftercare service. It was to be the complete, miniature, ideal *hospital and clinic*, with a bright energetic board-certified psychiatrist, two traditional Academy of Certified Social Workers, a psychologist, a head nurse with a complete nursing staff, a group of rehabilitation counselors, and a contingent of mental health program workers.

This last group was supposed to be the *new* human service workers but they were regarded with much suspicion by the rest of the staff. As there was no clearly defined role for most of the traditional staff, social workers, nurses, and psychologists, they were anxious about what it was these new people were supposed to do. It took nearly a year of infighting and a lot of staff turnover for the clinical treatment group to turn its attention to the community. The philosophy espoused by the agency director was that of providing short-term crisis-intervention services in the community, with the zone center itself being the link between the people and agencies of the community and the state department of mental health. Unfortunately the director was more scholarly than intuitive, more trusting of the staff's ability to accept the necessity for the programs to take priority over professional territorial imperatives and bureaucracy-building. Perhaps with time, the efficacy of the human services approach would have proved itself and prevailed, but early in the implementation of the decision-making machinery in the organization, the director incorporated some personnel from a small, existing, state-supported children's service agency. The half dozen members of this agency were professional elitists of each of the major disciplines who, in developing their careers, had completely accepted the medical-Freudian approach. Early in the development of the zone center, these professionals made themselves indispensable to the director; they gained control of the flow of information to and from him. They isolated the director and prevented or delayed the implementing of service programs. Within two years the director sensed that it was time to return to his scholarly pursuits at a prestigious medical school.

With his departure, control of the agency rapidly shifted to the traditional professionals. The friction this brought to the agency gradually drove away the more innovative pragmatists to other states and agencies. However, the agency *was* eventually able to get out into the community. It stopped the flow of patients to the state hospital and kept a lot of professionals employed. But its own research demonstrated that in spite of the high operating costs and the resources in manpower, materials and accomodations, they were not able to do any better job than the state hospitals. The agency's recidivism rate was just as high and it took just as long to return a patient to society. In addition, while the agency had stopped sending so many patients to the state hospitals, it had been forced to develop its own facilities for housing and dealing with its long-term patients, for whom they developed a new label, the *sub-acute*. It would seem that much of the agency's problems stemmed from an early decision to use its available mental health manpower traditionally rather than take the opportunity to develop and implement their human services manpower. Organizationally, the agency kept its small contingent of human service-oriented workers at the bottom of the career ladder in positions with low salary and little decision-making authority. This, of course, left the best (money, status, authority) to the traditional professionals, professionals who have taken on the coloration of innovators in order to maintain the status quo.

The State Hospital

An existing, large state mental hospital was also given a mandate to change, but it was expected to proceed with little new funding, buildings, or equipment. The mandate was: (1) primary responsibility for providing mental health services to two large catchment areas; (2) provide back-up service to two additional areas while a new mental health zone center began to operate; (3) provide service to a large geriatric population in addition to developing a network of community-based facilities for the elderly; (4) upgrade a moderate-sized children's and adolescents' program; (5) add an adult mental retardation program which was to accept patients from the state schools for the mentally retarded; (6) reduce an enormous population of long-term patients.

211

If the hospital was to make any progress, it was clearly going to have to be a bootstrap operation. By and large, the staff was oriented toward custodial care; the professional staff was primarily involved with individual counseling; and the hospital's training program focused primarily on a nursing school and departmentalized professional development.

As the hospital was staggering under the impact of the job ahead, one of the authors of this book—Walter Fisher—began looking about for alternate ways to deploy the existing manpower. It was immediately apparent that much valuable time and energy were being wasted through the departmentalized structure of the organization's response to the myriad problems and liabilities of its patients. The patient was being divided up physically and psychologically for treatment. The psychiatric aide had primary responsibility for his day-to-day life. The doctor made sporadic medical checks on the patient, based largely on information from the aide. The psychologist made tests and measurements. The patient's family and friends were the responsibility of a social worker who sometimes had a 200-patient caseload. A rehabilitation counselor and an activity therapist completed the *therapeutic* regimen. This group of treatment specialists rarely came to a decision about anything, from a treatment plan to when a patient was ready for discharge.

What was needed was someone who could function as a mental health *generalist* (a person willing to do anything). But it was easier to identify the correct concept than to implement it. Implementation was a lengthy, painful process. Established departments and services, ranging from psychology to housekeeping, had to be dismantled and their personnel and duties reassigned to other programs. New training strategies and organizations had to be developed, which emphasized programmatic competence rather than body mechanics. Finally, after many lengthy state-level committee meetings and several years of delays, the new mental health generalist series was officially made available for the agency to use in redeploying its personnel. Until this new series was officially available, a small number of persons were accommodated in the mental health program worker series. This series, however, was only marginally useful, in that both the departments of personnel and mental health stringently applied the rules concerning who qualified and who did not. The primary usefulness of the classification was to allow a small-scale training endeavor and the recruitment of a few new people. Eventually employees were rewarded financially and organizationally for on-the-job competence, responsibility, and participation in inservice training programs.

It was the first time that the possibility had existed of rewarding a person for being able to perform the job *competently* instead of for his credentials. As the staff were encouraged to perform responsibly and competently, it became apparent that not only were the traditional professionals not as effective in this kind of economy, but that the formal preparation acquired in college, particularly at the graduate level, was sometimes a liability. The reasons behind this problem with schools and universities and our initial approaches to a solution will be explored later. The agency's success in meeting its programmatic responsibilities is due largely to deploying its personnel in a human service mode, with inservice training programs and organizational change.

In comparing the attempts to meet the new mandates for service, both the mental health zone center and the state hospital had to develop service programs on the basis of what their respective economies would allow. The mental health zone center had the resources to develop programs along traditional lines, while the state hospital, confronted by an expanding demand for service and with few new resources, had to come up with new solutions in the face of an institutional-level crisis. The human service worker was such a solution.

In contrast to the mental health zone centers with large budgets, the problems and demands placed on the state hospital for new services closely parallel the difficulties faced by society since the end of World War II. During this period, the large state mental hospitals have become the hunting ground for muckraking sociologists and anthropologists. August B. Hollingshead and Frederick C. Redlich [1965] have demonstrated the high degree of correlation between the factors of levels of social stratification, psychiatric disorders, and consequences for the individual. If a person is from an affluent background, the mental health crisis is usually successfully resolved with little in the way of lingering social stigma. If, on the other hand, he is poor, disadvantaged, and unfortunate enough to get involved with the typical mental health care delivery system, he may well be in for a lifetime of unresolved problems and a career of mental illness.

213

SOCIAL STRATIFICATION AND PSYCHIATRIC DISORDERS*
by August B. Hollingshead and Frederick C. Redlich

One of the most signigicant large-scale social studies in "mental illness" ever undertaken was begun by the above authors in 1950 in the New Haven, Connecticut area. This is a brief report of three major findings: (1) There is a relationship between the incidence of mental illness and social class—the incidence is higher in the lower class; (2) There is a relationship between type of mental illness and social class—neuroses tend to occur in the upper classes, psychoses tend to occur in the lower classes; (3) There is a relationship between type of care or treatment received and social class—people in the upper classes receive care which is based upon our most up-to-date notions, those in the lower classes receive largely custodial care.

Perhaps the most disturbing finding and at the same time the one which most dramatically and convincingly illustrates the social nature of "mental illness" is the revelation that people in different social classes receive markedly different care even though their *behavior*–labeled many times as mental illness—*has been the same.*

The classes of citizens involved in the study:

Class I. This stratum is composed of wealthy families whose wealth is often inherited and whose heads are leaders in the community's business and professional pursuits. Its members live in those areas of the community generally regarded as "the best." The adults are college graduates, usually from famous private institutions, and almost all families are listed in the New Haven *Social Directory*. In brief, these people occupy positions of high social prestige.

Class II. Adults in this stratum are almost all college graduates; the males occupy high managerial positions; many are engaged in the lesser-ranking professions. These families are well-to-do, but there is no substantial inherited or acquired wealth. Its members live in the "better" residential areas; about half of the families belong to lesser-ranking private clubs, but only 5 percent of Class II families are listed in the New Haven *Social Directory*.

*From Ohmer Milton, ed., *Behavior disorders, perspectives and trends*, New York, Lippincott, 1965.

Class III. This stratum includes the vast majority of small pro-prietors, white-collar office and sales workers, and a considerable number of skilled manual workers. Adults are predominately high school graduates, but a considerable percentage have attended business schools and small colleges for a year or two. They live in "good" residential areas; less than 5 percent belong to private clubs, but they are not included in the *Social Directory*. Their social life tends to be concentrated in the family, the church, and the lodge.

Class IV. This stratum consists predominately of semi-skilled factory workers. Its adult members have finished the elementary grades, and those under 35 have generally completed high school. *Its members comprise almost one-half of the community*, and their residences are scattered over wide areas. Social life is centered in the family, the neighborhood, the labor union, and public places.

Class V. Occupationally, Class V adults are overwhelmingly semi-skilled factory hands and unskilled laborers. Educationally, most adults have not completed the elementary grades. The families are concentrated in the "tenement" and "cold-water flat" areas of New Haven. Only a small minority belong to organized community institutions. Their social life takes place in the family flat, on the street, or in neighborhood social agencies.

SELECTED FINDINGS

Table. I.
Distribution of Normal and Psychiatric Population by Social Class

Social Class	Normal Population		Psychiatric Population	
	number	percent	number	percent
I	358	3.1	19	1.0
II	926	8.1	131	6.7
III	2,500	22.0	260	13.2
IV	5,256	46.0	758	38.6
V	2,037	17.8	723	36.8
Unknown	345	3.0	72	3.7
Total	11,422	100.0	1,963	100.0

Table II.
Distribution of Neuroses and Psychoses by Social Class

	Neuroses		Psychoses	
Social Class	number	percent	number	percent
I	10	52.6	9	47.4
II	88	67.2	43	32.8
III	115	44.2	145	55.8
IV	175·	23.1	583	76.9
V	61	8.4	662	91.6
Total	449		1,442	

Table III
Comparison of the Distribution of the Normal Population with Schizophrenics by Class

	Normal Population		Schizophrenics	
Social Class	number	percent	number	percent
I	358	3.2	6	.7
II	926	8.4	23	2.7
III	2,500	22.6	83	9.8
IV	5,256	47.4	352	41.6
V	2,037	18.4	383	45.2
Total	11,077	100.0	847	100.0

Table IV
Distribution of the Principal Types of Therapy by Social Class

	Psychotherapy		Organic Therapy		No Treatment	
Social Class	number	percent	number	percent	number	percent
I	14	73.7	2	10.5	3	15.8
II	107	81.7	15	11.4	9	6.9
III	136	52.7	74	28.7	48	18.6
IV	237	31.1	288	37.1	242	31.8
V	115	16.1	234	32.7	367	51.2
Total	609		613		669	

Another report which shows the arbitrary classification of mental illness was conducted by M.H. Brenner [1967]. In a study of economic change and patterns of mental hospitalization, he has shown that fluctuations in the economy adversely affect the rate of hospitalization. These findings have led to a new spirit of consumerism among persons needing care. Increasingly, newspapers, legislators, and various federal agencies have led probes, asked questions, and withheld funds. Much of this activity is self-serving; for example, newspapers want increased circulation. But there is genuine public interest about how their money is being spent and what services are being provided. Such developments as county referendum boards, which are supported by citizens voluntarily increasing their taxes, are demanding and getting action in determining the operations of such things as mental health clinics and workshops. These agencies are comparable to school boards in operation and voter interest.

In the private sector, nationally recognized care-givers such as Thomas Szasz [1961] have raised questions about whether there really is such a phenomenon as mental illness or if, in fact, mental illness has not been *manufactured* by the system itself. Dr. Szasz has raised the consumer issue by making an analogy between haircutting and psychiatry: if you don't like the haircut, go to another barber. He feels that psychiatry should be on a completely voluntary basis. If you feel you aren't getting the kind of personal growth experiences you are paying for, you should find another counselor.

Robert Agranoff and Walter Fisher ("Decision Making in Mental Health") have raised the issue of accountability in an attempt to acquaint people with what are often the real basis for decisions. The foundation of mental health care is being shaken and questioned much as are other social institutions today.

Institutions In Decline

In order to put the decline and dysfunction of the traditional social institutions in perspective, we will briefy examine another kind of institution, which in many ways is closely related to the mental health industry.

For years, education, especially graduate training, has gone unquestioned. The skills of the professors and objectives of the courses went unchallenged. Few asked if the learning experience was leading to demonstrable competence on the job. Few considered the possibility that the schools were not doing their job and might be gradually becoming out of step with the real world. This is in fact what has happened, not only with the schools, but in many of the other previously unassailable institutions of our culture. Marshall McLuhan [1964] has suggested that with the advent of electronic media, information input, for the first time in history, is higher outside the classroom than inside and that the student must postpone his education every time he enters the classroom.

Technology and practice in most areas of competence are expanding more rapidly outside the university than within it. One of the authors had this pointed up very sharply a few years ago when he had an opportunity to spend several days at an inpatient crisis-intervention service which was affiliated with a medical school. The clinic was operated on the basis of very short-term hospitalization, using a combination of catharsis, chemotherapy, and problem-solving. One floor above was the psychiatric training center, which from time to time used the crisis-intervention service as a referral point for obtaining subjects on which the psychiatrist interns could practice. One morning the author attended a problem-solving session at the crisis-intervention program, which was attempting to patch up a young man who periodically got in trouble with the police. Every attempt was made to link him with other ways to occupy his spare time and gain socialization skills, all outside the service agency.

Following this session, the author was invited to the medical school upstairs to sit in on a session in which the *house analyst* would demonstrate his skill in working with children. The case that morning was a first grader displaying the classic symptoms of becoming upset when faced with the prospect of going off to school. The mother came in first and said she felt the problem was primarily that of helping her child feel more comfortable about going to school. To the mother's misfortune, the analyst was unwilling to accept this simple view of the problem; before the mother and child left, he had succeeded in initiating a long-term contract to explore the dynamics of the family and the mother's own unresolved feelings of frustration. Wondering how these two operations could be tolerated under one roof and feeling more rapport with the director of the crisis-intervention service, the author returned to ask him. When told what had happened, the director swore under his breath and said that when the interns came to work there, he had to spend a couple of weeks with them to *straighten them out* so they wouldn't damage too many innocent people. Here was an educational institution acutely behind the times in relation to the competence and skills demonstrated by the agency in the field.

An institution, either as a physical entity (a hospital) or as a cultural phenomenon (such as the family) is essentially a complex system for managing and expediting human behavior. This works only as long as the rules and procedures of the institution are actually expeditious for people. As the needs of most people affiliated in some way with an institution change, one of two things can happen: the institution changes to accommodate the new needs of the people it is organized to serve, or it becomes perceived as a regressive gatekeeper whose mission is to cause people trouble. At that point people will either quietly abandon the institution or openly rebel. Because of the inertia inherent in an institution, it is difficult for it to easily change; it will do so only in a crisis. This is just what has happened to many institutions in the past decade.

A period of great change, when many different forces are struggling to reorder priorities, is also a period in which institutional crises affect almost everyone. Most people are struggling to cope with several crises simultaneously. Nearly everyone is vulnerable. Most who seem to be making it are doing so only by maintaining a precarious balance of the forces and priorities in their lives. Never has the old concept of homeostasis had a more difficult time. We are living in a time when at any given moment, a person or family who feel in no danger can be thrown into crisis and need immediate help.

Summary

In this chapter we described the human service model as being pragmatic, problem-solving, brief, and as being universal with regard to persons and their problems. These characteristics have been developed in response to human needs at a time when the resources of time and money are limited.

219

The human service model has been traced through its development in several agencies which were called on to meet many new responsibilities while solving already existing problems and meeting day-to-day demands. We suggested that as institutions become increasingly out of touch with change, they become ineffectual, empty gatekeepers. It is usually only in the midst of a crisis that an institution will try a new alternative. Today, many social institutions, including mental health, are in the midst of a crisis. Most are struggling to find new and useful alternatives. The human service model is the kind of approach that is most useful as the demands for service increase and as resources become more limited.

Chapter 15 *The Human Service Model: Systems*

I n this chapter and the next we will focus on the various beliefs, assumptions, ideologies, and philosophies of the human service model. The list of items for Chapter 15 and 16 has been limited to eight, not because it is all-inclusive or because it contains all of the important *truths*. The list contains those items with which the authors have had first-hand experience Rather than being developed in a think-tank situation, they have evolved through problem-solving processes and real situations. Each grew out of situations we encountered in treatment programs, training and development projects, and working situations with colleges and universities. As each of the beliefs, assumptions, ideologies, and philosophies is presented, we will put it in perspective by giving examples and case histories, discussing its significance in the human service model, and briefly describing its impact. The items included in Chapter 15 are:

1. The immediate, major problem in the field is to establish a meaningful economy, effective evaluation, and true accountability.

2. An understanding has to be developed that there are many causes of maladaptive behavior and they require multiple approaches.

3. Program primacy which meets the needs, problems, and crises of the community and patients is a major priority issue.

In Chapter 15 the primary focus will be on the concerns of human services at the systems level, while in Chapter 16, issues related to attitudes, manpower, and training will be examined.

NUMBER 1: The immediate, major problem in the field is to establish a meaningful economy, effective evaluation, and true accountability. In struggling with these issues, it will be helpful to briefly consider how the economy of any system operates. In the business world, industry, stores, and services, while tied to the general economy, have their own economic resources which demand programming, planning, and budgeting. This takes place either formally, with management and cost-accounting departments, or informally, with the owner-operator sitting down after the store closes and taking stock of where he is and what plans need to be made to satisfy his customers. Of course, any mistakes in planning will be reflected in the economy of the company. If there are too many mistakes, the company will suffer and the customer will take his business elsewhere. The *theory* behind this is that of free enterprise. Who can deliver the best service or merchandise at the least cost will be the winner in this economic survival of the fittest.

There have been many exceptions to the free enterprise system in our culture. The exceptions occur whenever some necessary commodity or service can in theory, be provided best by a publicly owned monopoly such as the utility and telephone companies. In other situations the exception is justified on the basis of controlling the quality of the service and the competence of the practitioner by such organizations as labor unions (plumbers, carpenters, electricians) and professional organizations such as the American Medical Association. Sometimes these limitations on the free enterprise system lead to greater efficiency and improved public welfare, on other occasions they do not. When they do not, it is extremely difficult for the individual consumer to get redress from these various public trusts and monopolies. It is only recently that a new spirit of consumerism has begun to take action. In the last few years, citizen action groups have formed and they have started to exert pressure and demand changes for better products and services.

The mental health service is one of the public trusts which has not gone untouched by these developments. There have been many calls from consumers and taxpayers for agencies to define their economies in terms of their economic resources (tax money) and how the money will be used (programming, planning, and budgeting). (See J.B. Alexander and J.L. Messal [1972].) The considerations raised by the issues of economy, evaluation, and accountability are: What are the priorities for allocating the resources of the mental health care system? Are these the priorities of the users or of the agency itself? What are the operationally defined boundaries of the system? What are the goals and philosophy of the service agency? How have the system's goals and philosophy been implemented? Have the agency's goals been achieved in keeping with the priority of the user?

Such questions must be considered by staff who try to establish an economy, evaluation, and accountability. They become particularly important when answers are sought beyond easy generalizations such as *to provide a humane milieu in which meaningful, therapeutic interventions can occur.* While such an objective appears on the surface to be a worthwhile goal, it raises more questions than it answers. If the student, as an experiment, sent out such a statement and asked various service program directors, first, if they agreed with it, and second, "What is a humane milieu?" we are sure every director would answer yes to the first question and give varying answers to the second. One service's program director might stress physical cleanliness in a humane milieu, while another might stress socialization activities. Also, we would expect that nearly always, members of the same service team would not agree on what the important features of a humane milieu are.

The point of this search for answers is that service program directors, team leaders, and individual service team members should define operationally what they mean, so they can avoid seeking competing goals. Their goals may include discharging six patients a month, getting all the residents off a ward for two hours a day, or making aftercare visits to all patients discharged or termi-

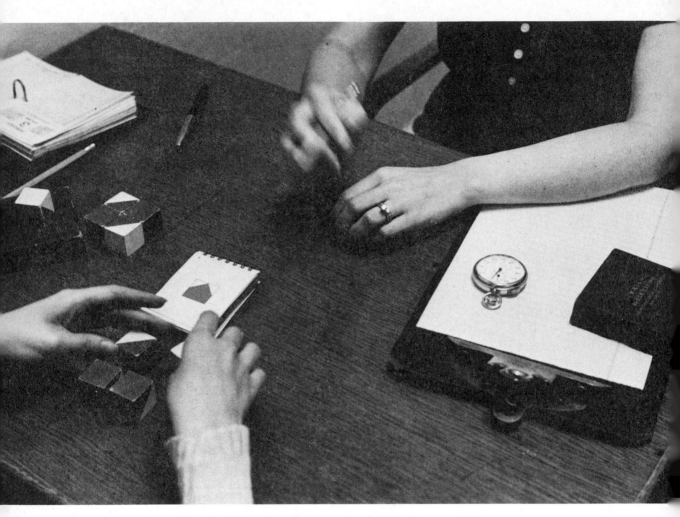

Meaningful testing, as a part of rehabilitation, can help establish an effective economy so essential to the working human service model. (Photo by Inge Morath, courtesy Magnum.)

nated in the past two weeks. The service team might also develop goals for individual patients such as, "Martha will make her bed every morning, go to her activity group, and use a knife and fork to eat her meals" or, "George will pay his own way in therapy." These goals have two immediate benefits: the staff may for the first time agree on what it is they are trying to accomplish on either a pro-grammatic level or an individual level; and operationalized goals allow the team to objectively quantify their success. For example, if the team's period of accounting covers a full week, they can demon-strate that they were able to get 76 percent of the patients off the ward for two hours a day or that the team was able to make only 18 percent of their aftercare visits. With this kind of information, a treatment team can articulate what services are being provided and what goals are being achieved. If, on investigation, they or some other administrator or legislator asks questions about what the treatment team is doing, they can tell him, based on an objective evaluation of their program. If the treatment team is not delivering appropriate or adequate service to the patients, several things can be done. First, their economy can be expanded; more staff can be hired, more equipment can be purchased, more training be given. It may be that the economy cannot be expanded or that some services such as a complicated group therapy program or social event will have to be scrapped. For example, it may be more important to get the patients involved in a daily job of dusting, making beds, and emptying ash trays than to have an individual 25-minute counseling session. Ob-viously dusting is not necessarily more important than counseling. We simply mean that the agency must decide on its priorities. An agency may not have a Mayo Brothers economy, so priorities must be established so the essential services can be provided. In this way, the human service mental health field can establish a *meaningful* economy, *effective* evaluation, and *true* accountability.

The establishment of all this is essential to everyone. By its very nature, the typical agency's economy does not allow for complicated, long-term care in which the patient is institutionalized. As is pointed out in Part III, there are not enough resources to go around if we are to utilize a medical-Freudian-hospital-disease-cure model in the public sector.

NUMBER 2: An understanding has to be developed that there are many causes of maladaptive behavior and they require multiple ap-

225

proaches. The belief that there are many causes of maladaptive behavior in the individual is a radical departure from the medical model, which endorses the identification and cataloging of symptoms and relating them to the disease in a direct cause-and-effect relationship. The result was to control symptoms through physical and chemical assaults upon the unfortunates who found their way into mental hospitals. Unfortunately, merely controlling maladaptive behavior does not solve a person's problems in terms of making him more adaptive or better able to cope with his situation. Controlling symptoms is society's way of isolating that part of a person's personality that makes people uncomfortable.

When Tommy, a second grader, becomes disruptive in the classroom, the solution, according to the medical model, is not to find a different kind of classroom, one that meets Tommy's needs. Tommy may be very bright and has become bored with the classroom work, or he may have problems at home and cannot concentrate, or he may be simply hyperactive. The solution to his disruptive behavior usually does not develop from the child's perspective, but instead from teacher and counselor frustration. They often view the situation not as to how it can be altered—what are alternative solutions for helping Tommy cope successfully?—but rather, how to use a ready-made, expedient solution based on a simple diagnosis sanctioned by their colleagues and society. Their strategy is to *control* Tommy's behavior.

The medical profession, among its many accomplishments, has come up with effective measures for controlling symptoms. Initially, it may suggest that Tommy is hyperactive (simple diagnosis) and that the symptoms can be controlled with drugs (treatment). The drugs should quickly remove the disruptive portion of Tommy's behavior (cure). If they don't, the medical profession prescribes more powerful drugs. If all else fails, they can resort to psychosurgery (lobotomy). Unfortunately for Tommy, the teacher, and even the doctor, the entire process has effects other than the chemical effect on Tommy's body. For Tommy, the experience is a nonsolution, in that it did nothing about his basic problem. For the teacher, the nonsolution is a lesson in suppressing disruptive behavior with the help of the family doctor. The experience did little to show those involved how to look for the many possible causes of the problem, and no experience in providing alternatives to the classroom situation in which Tommy was having trouble. In addition, for Tommy it has brought a diagnosis of hyperactivity—or minimal brain damage—which will follow him throughout his life and which can always be referred to if behavioral problems arise later.

In Chapter 2, Norris Hansell's [1970] and A.H. Maslow's [1954] need motivation systems were discussed. Both writers spell out the many factors in a person's life that must be considered when looking for the cause of strange behavior and trying to determine what there might be in his life that needs support and development. A more detailed listing of Hansell's need system is comprised of seven inter-related subsystems.

Hansell's Need System

A human being must have available and be able to incorporate water, food, oxygen, new experiences, and information. The needs of this subsystem revolve around the individual's environment and his ability to interact with it. The commodities necessary for him within this subsystem are generally available in our culture, and special concern is usually given only to infants and the very elderly who may have physical difficulty in getting what they need. There are, however, several other groups of people who may not be getting what they need, especially new experiences and information. These people are the residents of mental hospitals and sheltered-care facilities, housewives, school children, persons in general hospitals, and residents of the new high-rise, low-income apartment houses, which replace slum dwellings. The possibility exists for persons in these groups to suffer from an environment depleted of experience and information stimulation.

The second need subsystem of the individual is having available, and being able to participate in intimate relationships. This need is usually thought of as being met within the boundaries of the family. But there are many for whom a family does not exist or if it does, is not working very well. Recent data about the divorce rate in Chicago suggest that some 40 percent of the marriages are so intolerable that they are formally ended by divorce proceedings in spite of the high financial and emotional costs. Other marriages continue legally but provide little in the way of satisfactory relationships on an intimate level. The reasons for this are many. Husbands, wives, and children may be truly incompatible due to changes of interest and values over several years or it may be that there has recently developed or has

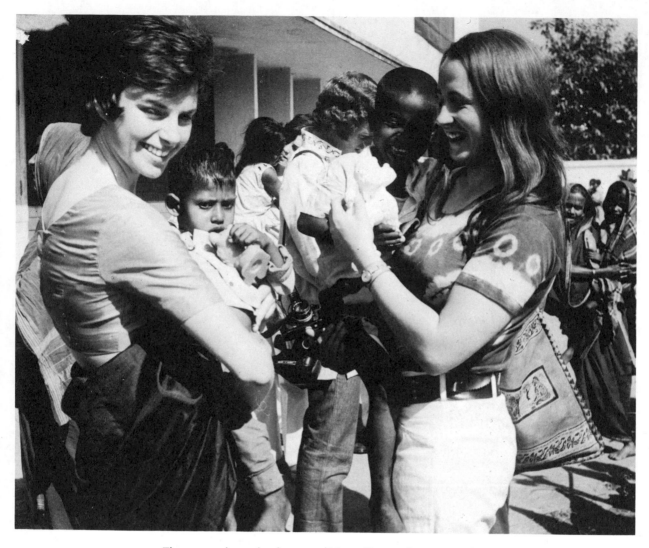

The second need subsystem (Hansell's need system) of the individual is having available, and being able to participate in, intimate relationships. Kathy Clark and nurse Joan O'Hanlon, Children's Hospital, Dacca. (Photo courtesy. Holy Ghost Fathers and Father Aloysius Dempsey.)

always existed a difficulty for one or more members of the family to relate comfortably on this level. For persons living outside a family unit, they, of course, have to develop different patterns of relationships which will handle this need.

The third need subsystem is that of having a sense of belonging to some kind of peer group. These peer group relationships may be developed through work-connected relationships, affiliation with some kinds of organized groups such as churches or lodges, or they may develop spontaneously within the context of the neighborhood. There are any number of groups of persons for whom peer group relationships are either unavailable or the person is unable to participate in them satisfactorily. Some of these situations involve elderly persons whose friends have died, families of persons who must move frequently because of job demands, patients in hospitals, and people who live in new high-rise ghettos. They all acutely need meaningful, ongoing relationships with groups of people who respect one another.

The fourth need subsystem involves a feeling of identity for the individual, a feeling that gives him an idea, not only of what and who he is, but that he is a worthwhile human being. Feelings of a cherishable identity arise from mutual feelings of respect between a person and the people he encounters, from ideas about the acceptability of his physical characteristics and how he takes care of himself, and a sense of being able to cope with the majority of daily problems that arise.

The fifth need subsystem is that of an ongoing role. Roles involve being a milkman, banker, mother, teacher, or student. The role a person takes is important to his maintaining his dignity. This occurs when the person's role performance is at an acceptable level in relation to a real or perceived standard. In other words, he feels he is doing a reasonably good job as a milkman, housewife, or student—or several of these roles combined. Without the opportunity or capacity to perform adequately in a role, a person feels no sense of dignity. Persons who have difficulty meeting this need successfully include housewives whose children have grown up and left home, recently retired workers, long-term patients leaving mental health facilities, transients, migrant workers, persons whose jobs have been eliminated because of automation, and those who have been fired because of incompetence.

The sixth need subsystem is for the person to be tied securely to the cash economy, through a salary, retirement program, public aid, member of a family, or inherited wealth. The person must feel that he has the financial resources to acquire shelter, food, health services, and many other essentials. Examples of persons who do not have this capacity include patients in mental hospitals, prisoners in jail, persons without salable job skills, and the elderly.

The seventh need subsystem involves the person who can make decisions based on some kind of comprehensive system of meaning. That is, the person has developed a system of priorities for making difficult choices between competing options. It does not matter so much whether he has all of the right priorities; it only matters that he can make the necessary decisions. Those who may have difficulty meeting this need are the elderly, who are often senile, confused, and disoriented in crises, or perhaps those new to our culture who are trying to adapt and are not sure what is right and wrong in our system.

The subsystems listed must all be functioning adequately or a person will not be able to survive. Not only are there many possibilities for failure, but the failures tend to involve each other and lead to the collapse of the person's ability to cope. For example, the person who is experiencing difficulty with his job for any of the reasons given will not only suffer a loss of dignity, he will suffer malfunctions in terms of his link to the cash economy, as well as problems with his relationships on both a peer level and an intimate level. One subsystem failure is almost always compounded by the breakdown of other subsystems.

When the human service worker attempts to intervene with the individual who has voluntarily or involuntarily come for service, he should always look for multiple breakdowns in the person's capacity to cope. There is no one problem the solving of which will make everything all right. The person in crisis or the person being returned to the community from prison, the hospital, or other kinds of institutions needs a broadly defined package of services and supports. For example, if he has become depressed and attempts suicide following a break-up in his marriage, it is not enough to hospitalize, medicate, and provide counseling services. This person will need a broad package of services in order to reenter the community. He may need a job, new friends, a new place to live, someone to share experiences with, perhaps a readjustment of his value system, and certainly some help with his identity. If he is not provided with this help, he will not be able to survive in the community and will likely revert to his earlier condition.

NUMBER 3: Program primacy which meets the needs, problems, and crises of the community and patients is a major priority issue. Programs must be developed which meet the needs of the community and the various human service users, rather than programs that are harmonious with the needs and training of the care-giver. One of the basic, and unfortunate, tendencies of human nature is an unwillingness to let go of ideas and notions in which a lot of time and energy have been invested. This is, in fact, what has happened to many professionals, psychiatrists, social workers, psychologists, community mental health workers, community organizers, and behavior modification experts.

Whenever mental health workers invest a lot of their resources in learning the mechanics and technology of the system—be it Sigmund Freud, Carl Rogers, Clark Hull, or Gerald Caplan—they are bound to see every situation as fitting that mold perfectly. It is almost as if they themselves went into crisis by having their comprehensive system of meaning violated. They have been highly trained in one school of thought and can make decisions only within that framework. This tendency is especially dangerous and non-productive when the professional therapist's particular treatment model does not fit the model agreed upon by the rest of the team. This leads to fractionalization of the program's problem-solving resources and inhibits its effectiveness in getting service to those who need it.

Such situations highlight the need for program and organizational development efforts on the part of the treatment teams, in which their goals and objectives are clearly and operationally defined. This sort of public accountability helps individual members of the treatment delivery system work toward agreed-upon goals. They should be conversant with the objectives of the system, the contingency plans for meeting these objectives, and how their role is a part of the total system. With the advent of more information, fewer people would be disenfranchised from the mainstream of thought and activity and could then decide whether they wanted to be a participant in the system. The institution could expect increased use of its resources for meeting goals of various groups to which the facility is accountable.

Summary

The first belief discussed in this chapter was that of establishing a meaningful economy, effective evaluation, and true accountability. We presented a kind of constitutional framework for the student of the human services, by which he may demand and make effective evaluations and bring true accountability to his own efforts, the efforts of others, and any program he may find himself involved in. Persons affiliated with the human service model should welcome an accounting and testing of their programs. In this way, services provided will always be in line with the problems and concerns of *all* the people in our quickly evolving culture.

Chapter 16 *The Human Service Model: Manpower*

In this second chapter dealing with the beliefs, assumptions, ideologies, and philosophies of the human service model, we will focus on the remaining aspects of the model, those having to do with staff attitudes and development of manpower resources:

4. Increase the available manpower to meet the expanding contingencies of the human services user.

5. Widen the perspective of the treatment staff with regard to service models, delivery systems, intervention, and prevention models.

6. The ultimate criterion for delivering service should be competence.

7. Services must constantly be brought into line with the needs of the users.

8. Mental health services are the right of all members of the

community. There should be some treatment for everybody rather than polarized treatment patterns, with services available for everyone, everywhere, at all times.

NUMBER 4: Increase the available manpower to meet the expanding contingencies of the human services user. Increasing the available manpower resources basically will involve the following opportunities: the creation of new professions such as the human service worker and the mental health generalist; the retraining of existing professions to fill new roles, thus enabling them to deliver new kinds of services; the identification of persons who as a result of their special social roles have therapeutic capabilities.

The first two sources for expanding the mental health manpower involve the development of new inservice training programs (Fisher, Mehr, and Truckenbrod [1973]), cooperative programs between educational institutions and service agencies, and a new public education model which would encourage energetic persons with pragmatic problem-solving ability to seek careers in the human services. We deal with these issues later in this chapter and now explore the third source for new manpower.

The third source will grow out of the process of identifying persons who, as a result of their special social roles, have abilities in therapy. This is, of course, a new, wide-open, untapped option. Listed below are a few examples of persons whose social roles place them in a position where they can provide support, commence the problem-solving process, and initiate the linking into the human service network.

Policemen. Front-line crisis intervention agents. Make decisions about appropriateness of different kinds of treatment. Give people advice on legal questions and resolve disputes.

Grade school teachers. Monitor ongoing development of children's general health and well-being. Direct families to various services needed, such as children and family-counseling services. Make suggestions about special learning programs for parents and children.

Bartenders. Could make referrals to alcohol and drug abuse treatment centers independently or in cooperation with police.

Bankers. Give advice on how different kinds of financial problems can be handled. Give credit advice and provide fiscal planning.

Professional tradesmen such as plumbers, carpenters, and electricians. Could run classes on how low-income persons can save money by making necessary home repairs themselves.

High school and college teachers. Could design and teach courses which would upgrade job skills and income potential of poverty-level persons in the community.

Retired men and women. Could set up and help run day-care centers for young children and the very elderly, helping make both periods of life more meaningful.

From these examples the student can get an idea of the dimension and kinds of human services needed by the members of the community. Many fall in the category of prevention and would therefore affect the rate of crises in the community positively. To be truly effective, a *bank* of persons, with all sorts of therapy roles for specific situations and problems should be created. This would permit a precise kind and quality of human service to be made available for the wide range of human problems arising in communities.

NUMBER 5: Widen the perspective of treatment staff with regard to service models, delivery systems, intervention, and prevention models. Closely following the belief that there are many causes of maladaptive behavior is the belief that service delivery systems must be given a wider perspective in intervening in maladaptive behavior and symptoms, as well as preventing their occurrence. A corollary is that as many personal growth experiences as possible must be made available to the individual in trouble if there is to be any hope of significantly involving him in a process that will help him overcome his difficulty. The following examples demonstrate how services can be expanded. One concerns a ward program in a large state hospital and the other a hypothetical, but necessary, expansion of the concept and practice of community mental health in a community clinic. In both examples we will attempt to draw your attention to ways of increasing services to people by making use of available resources, changing patterns of communication, and developing new staff expectations.

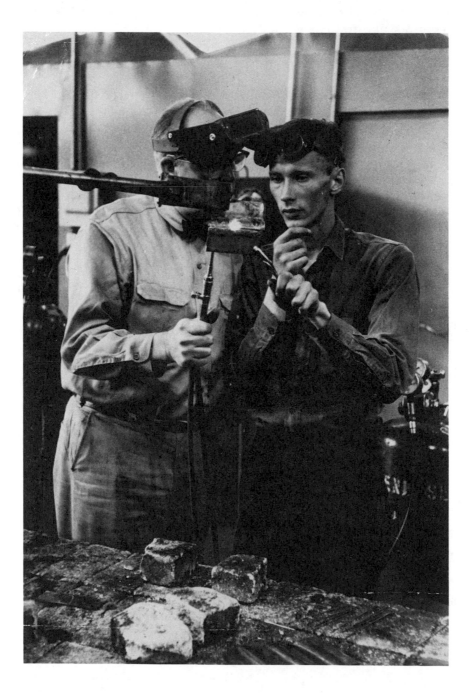

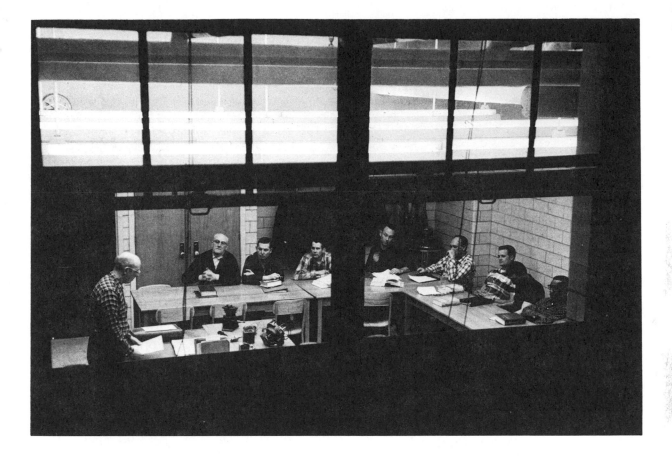

An important phase of the human service rehabilitation program is the training and retraining of individuals by qualified instructors. (Photos by Wayne Miller, courtesy Magnum.)

A Ward Treatment Program

Several years ago, as the result of a hospital-wide reorganization, one of the wards in a large state hospital was faced with the responsibility for 65 long-term, chronic, female patients. This particular group was the inpatient bottom of the barrel from two catchment areas.

At the time of the reorganization, the ward was referred to as a *catchment back-up service,* which meant that the ward took the leftover patients (roughly half) who were admitted to a mental health zone center. In theory, the state hospital back-up service got the extra admissions on a random basis; patients admitted to the state hospital were supposed to be similar to those the zone center kept on the basis of severity of problems, age, race, and social resources. What actually happened was that a clinical reason was found to justify transferring the more *damaged* people to the state hospital. The reason usually given was that these people would benefit from a longer stay in the hospital.

There were three different services. There was an admissions program, which sought to treat quickly as many as possible of the new admissions from the zone center in an intensive treatment program. In a second program there was an attempt to use group therapy and group activity strategies for longer-term, but more coherent, patients. The third program involved three wards, two female and one male. These wards housed the leftover, chronic patients from the catchment areas and whoever else happened to be in the state hospital. These were the patients with the gravest prognosis. The 65 patients in one of the female wards that will be described were the most unlikely and unappetizing group of humanity the authors have ever seen herded together. They were without any redeeming social values. They had nothing to which the staff could relate. Their average length of hospitalization was 27 years. Fully half were untidy and refused to wear anything. They had two basic drives (beyond eliminating wherever they stood)—eating and sleeping. The first time one of the authors saw this ward was shortly after he had started working at the hospital. He had to go to the ward to pick up some papers. Upon unlocking the door and entering the day room, he saw 35 or 40 faded, plastic, turquoise rocking chairs occupied by the old women, some smoking state-supplied tobacco, some ritualistically chanting and swearing. Sleeping patients, some naked and some in hospital gowns, were scattered around the room. The staff, of course, were huddled in the nurses' station reading magazines. After all, what could two psychiatric aides and an activity therapist do with this ward full of unwanted bodies.

Shortly after this, one of the authors was transferred to the ward along with two staff members. What was to be done? None of the staff had any particular skill or desire to rehabilitate the *super*-damaged product of 20 some years of snake-pit existence. There was little sense of mission about the challenge. Out of desperation, it was decided that three things had to be done immediately: (1) the door to the dormitory was to be locked to prevent the patients from sneaking back to bed to sleep; (2) the rocking chairs were to be traded to another ward for more suitable furnishing; and (3) a clothing room packed with discarded useless rags and junk was to be cleaned and made into office space.

When this had been done, the ward, staff and patients, while not ready to win any prizes for progress had been markedly restructured. There was a subtle change in the behavior of a few of the patients and a slight feeling of optimism on the part of the staff, which prompted further changes during the following year: housekeeping details, involving all of the staff and all of the patients, were initiated; a marginal activity program was begun; a patient-government was started (at first the patients had to be forced to attend); several of the patients were identified as having the potential to survive in the outside world; as the better patients were discharged, others spontaneously took their places as good patients and were also eventually discharged; a staff member started a *good-grooming group*, using donated tubes of lipstick, powder, a hairbrush, and a mirror; patients were literally and physically forced to leave the ward several times a week to go on *marches* or see the weekly movie on the hospital grounds; the staff no longer tolerated patients being undressed or untidy; all of the staff, including the psychiatric aides, were involved in writing progress reports, periodic reviews, and discharge notes—they all had a *caseload;* gradually the total number of patients was reduced to a manageable

239

number, which allowed the staff to work on the more complicated discharges requiring public-aid referrals, visits to nursing homes and sheltered-care facilities, and the restoration of civil rights for the legally incompetent; the artificial caste boundaries between the psychiatric aide and the rest of the staff began to break down, and communication and cooperation improved dramatically.

If at the end of that year a stranger had visited the ward, he would have been shocked at how awful the place looked and how sad the condition of the patients. But to those familiar with the ward, the changes were unbelievable and most encouraging. The change in the ward was a night to day kind of experience, not only for the patients, but also for the staff.

The staff's perspective of the kinds of services that would be useful and effective to the severely damaged patient had been widened. The service model was changed from that of a departmentalized, custodial model to one of a generalist human services model. This new human services approach attempted to incorporate the belief that human growth experiences could take place *throughout the day* and not just in traditional group therapy and counseling.

A Community Mental Health Clinic

Typically, the services provided to a community by its community mental health clinic are restricted to crisis intervention services, short-term counseling, and medication maintenance programs. This, of course, is a limited concept of the service that *could* be provided. In most cases, the local community mental health clinic does not provide even these limited services to all comers freely and nondiscriminatively. We know of several that discriminate against blacks, Chicanos, the poor, and other minority groups, choosing instead to serve the white middle class who can afford private treatment. For a community mental health clinic to be effective, several changes in perspective must occur:

● The community mental health clinic must remain oriented toward the *territorial* (geographic) approach. The authors feel this is the best delivery system.

● The clinic must not discriminate on the basis of age, sex, or particular problems and should operate on a "no decline option." This does not mean that the clinic should treat every patient directly. There will be times when potential patients can best be served by other agency programs in the community. These arrangements for linking should be worked out on a contractual basis, with the patient never being caught in the middle and thus lost from the treatment network. Programs should never be filled or closed. The waiting list should be abandoned, and as programs fill, the best patients should be discharged.

- Personnel responsible for the mental health care delivery system for the community should be sensitive to the idea that the community can be changed to support its citizens rather than isolating them.
- The community mental health delivery system should be organized to maintain continuity of treatment within the community—between the community and the clinic, and from the clinic back to the community.
- The importance of the screening, linking, and planning operation cannot be overly stressed. The clinic must establish contact with concerned relatives, neighbors, and other community agencies.
- Community programs should be developed as alternatives to residential care, for example, halfway houses, partial hospitalization, or visiting human service teams.
- With proper screening and linking, few should be isolated from the community. Service alternatives should be developed for every conceivable type of problem requiring human service, and the person in need should have easy access to them.
- The community mental health clinic should work with other service agencies, governmental groups, and citizens to develop programs that will prevent human service problems from reaching the crisis stage.

By applying these guidelines, our hypothetical community mental health clinic would achieve a wider perspective of its service model, delivery system, and intervention and prevention models.

In describing both service programs—the female ward in a large state hospital and the community mental health clinic—we have attempted to demonstrate the efficacy of designing and implementing treatment programs as broadly and innovatively as possible. In both programs, priority is placed on making the program workable

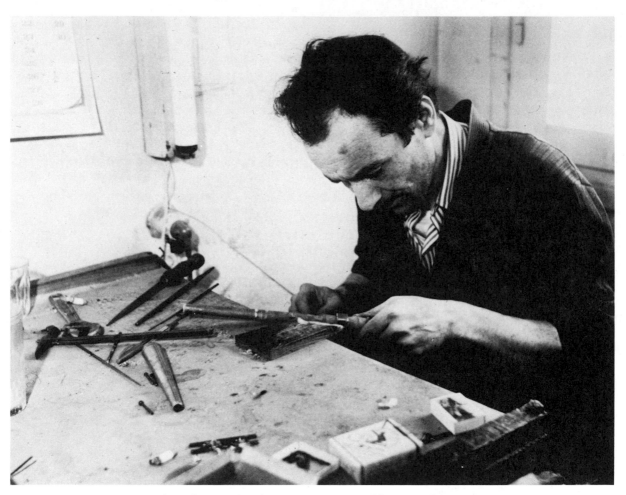

A loan from a social service agency enables an artisan to become self-sufficient. (Courtesy, Joint Distribution Committee.)

and oriented toward problem-solving, in an effort to find the system alternatives that work for the patient.

NUMBER 6: The ultimate criterion for delivering service should be competence. It is important to identify those skills that are necessary for delivering effective services to a wide variety of patients. The belief that the treatment staff's competence is crucial to the delivery of services must be seen within the context of the treatment program itself (Truckenbrod [1972]). That is, the staff must be competent in those skills directly related to the objectives of the treatment program. For example, if the program is oriented toward behavior modification, the skills of a highly trained psychoanalyst are irrelevant. The idea of competence, however, goes beyond the variable of training to include a personal-equation factor which has been characterized as a person's age, energy, and personality.

At one agency it has become standard practice to promote and assign responsibility to persons on the basis of personal experience, inservice training, and the personal-equation factor, which has led to greater success in picking and promoting a person than by merely looking at his credentials. This style of operation has led to the career ladder concept which endorses and validates promotions based on training and competence. There is a major drawback, however: those who moved up the career ladder through personal competence, but who lacked university credentials, were locked into the agency. Other mental health agencies would not allow such persons, regardless of ability, to transfer into their system at equivalent positions. As the authors explored this problem, two things became painfully apparent: (1) in the field of mental health and probably in most fields, university credentials are much more important than personal competence; and (2) certain job transfers are almost entirely based on university credentials. Clearly the best way to validate competence is to link it to college credits and degrees which are universally transferable and acceptable.

NUMBER 7: Services must constantly be brought into line with the needs of the users. If services are to remain relevant, it is crucial to link the users to the service agencies and the service agencies to the education system. The agencies have to monitor needs continually in order to adjust programs to these need systems. This belief has arisen out of the new spirit of consumerism that has occurred within the past decade. The public is becoming more and more interested in the delivery of goods and services by mental health facilities, as well as public services such as colleges and universities. Taxpayers and students are demanding that their courses and training provide them with relevant learning. Recent drops in university enrollment point to an expanding gap between the training provided by many traditional college departments and actual requirements in the field. Service agencies have found that it matters less what the new employee studied in college than his receptivity to new ideas and willingness to work toward program goals and objectives.

The dilemmas cited above have started to bring the service agencies and the universities together to form a more effective working relationship. This relationship is moving the institutions to accept the following themes in forming new kinds of interinstitutional relations:

Linking of academic credit with inservice training. Much university-level training is provided to employees of many types of agencies, but this training has generally been *creditless.* The system must be modified so that people also receive accreditation for their growth.

Provide degree programs which will yield vertical and horizontal mobility. Inservice training generally provides vertical mobility (a person can be promoted within a system). However, horizontal mobility (the ability to move between systems) while maintaining an equitable pay level, depends in our society on being credentialed by universities. The interagency network, as a goal, will provide accredited degrees which, in turn, will provide the certification.

Maximize utilization of previously economically and educationally disadvantaged entry-level persons. Upgrading of entry-level employees through training that is college-creditable and that focuses on new treatment processes will maximize the value of the employees to the agency.

Put the interdisciplinary-generalist concept into practice. The interdisciplinary-generalist approach seems more worthwhile, both economically and functionally, than training in narrow specialties.

Use training programs to develop new roles for employees in human service systems. In changing mental health delivery systems, training can be a valuable input in the development and implementation of new roles for human service workers.

Open the previously closed university system to the nonprofessional employee who has not typically made use of these systems. State hospital manpower, in many cases, consists of individuals who have had negative experiences in schooling and for whom the university ladder is unavailable psychologically, economically, or physically. The educational-relinking network is an attempt to provide an acceptable *schooling* format for these people.

Provide a screening-in entrance system rather than a screening-out system. Universities have traditionally screened out those who have not succeeded, in the usual sense, in their system. The network is committed to an open-door policy.

Develop systems for trainee support in the university system. As a corollary to the preceding point, screening-in necessitates the development of systems for remedial education and training, a trainee advocacy staff, financial support, and child care.

Develop a system where field staff and trainees can share in the design of college programs. The cry of *irrelevance* has arisen in the criticism of the university system. We feel that universities are at least 10 years behind service agencies in the material they teach; for example, most universities continue training in Rorschach techniques long after most agencies have recognized their irrelevance in day-to-day work. Agencies must have a stake in what is taught to the students who will someday be their employees. The education-relinking network provides a process in which this can be done.

Help the educational facilities in trying out a new role–the university as a means of overcoming alienation by relinking persons to a career ladder. In the past, universities have contributed to the alienation through elitist selection practices. A screening-in educational-relinking process is a new mode of functioning for the university.

Develop a system for authenticating and validating human growth experiences. We are convinced that many human experiences are educational growth experiences that can be authenticated to a sufficient degree to obtain college credit for the individual experiencing them.

These themes will help you define a more sensitive relationship between schools and service agencies, service agencies and their employees, and service agencies and taxpayer-citizen-consumers. The sensitivity not only will come to pass because of discussion and meetings but because of direct monetary support from taxes, tuition, and grants. There is a growing tendency for foundations to put funding in the hands of the consumer agency rather than give it directly to the educational facility. These changes, which are in the early phases of development, should change the atmosphere and direction of both education-training and the ability of an agency to provide services as the result of better employee competence.

NUMBER 8: Mental health services are the right of all members of the community. There should be some treatment for everybody rather than polarized treatment patterns, with services available for everyone, everywhere, at all times. At one point in the history of providing mental health services, there were two clearly defined systems, the services in the public sector and those in the private sector. The system one found oneself in was determined by one factor—ability to pay. If one had the money, he could buy fairly effective services. If he was poor, he would quickly find himself on a one-way trip to a career of chronic patienthood. A.B. Hollingshead and F.C. Redlich [1965], who have presented definitive data on this, concluded: "Perhaps the most disturbing findings and at the same time the one which most dramatically and convincingly illustrates the social nature of 'mental illness' is the revelation that people in different social classes receive markedly different care, even though their behavior——labeled many times as mental illness—*has been the same.*"

This whole style of thinking is obviously unacceptable in a civilized culture and does not fall into line with President John F. Kennedy's (1963) message to Congress in which he endorsed the notion that all citizens have a right to effective mental health services. In the ten years since President Kennedy put forth this mandate, there has been a lot of taxpayer money spent, but little to point to in terms of success. The reasons are many, not the least being that the mental health problem was greatly underestimated in size and complexity while the resources available to solve the problem were very much over-rated. The fact remains, however, that the problem still exists, and must be solved. The concept of a broadly conceived system of care delivery called the human services has defined the parameters of the problem and is beginning to exert its influence.

The human services model must establish new priorities for effective treatment for everyone, rich and poor alike, and at all places on an around the clock basis.

The new priorities must include a belief in the greatest possible continuity of treatment and the least isolation of patients from the service system. This means that when the patient enters the human services network, he must not be lost through the frustration of being put on a waiting list, having sloppy referral work linking him from one agency to another, or come to believe that no one is really interested in helping him solve his problems. They must be involved in action-oriented, problem-solving service. In order to meet the expanded needs for the services generated by such a treatment model, another important basic assumption must be implemented. Society has available to it a huge number of *growth experiences.* Schoolrooms, therapists' offices, community organizations, and new social institutions are only a portion of the possibilities. To make them available to the individual citizen in our society, a process must be developed in which we can identify and authenticate the experiences by which people grow and develop (Fisher, Mehr, and Truckenbrod [1973]).

Summary

In this chapter you have been exposed to three methods of increasing the available manpower to meet the expanding contingencies of the human service user—creating new professions such as the human service worker and the mental health generalist, retraining existing professions to fill new roles, and identifying those who, as a result of their special social roles, have therapeutic capabilities.

As a part of increasing service to the user, existing treatment staff must attempt to expand their ideas about what the essential components of treatment are and then act on them.

Another important factor in delivering service is the competence of the human service worker. The necessary competence for providing service must be identified, then ways to validate it must be established, probably through some type of university credentialing.

The services delivered must be continuously brought into line with the needs of the user, and the human service worker must be trained in relevant skills. Finally, mental health services are the right of all members of the community. There should be some treatment for everybody, rather than polarized treatment patterns, with services being available for everyone, everywhere, at all times.

Chapter 17 *The Organization of Human Service Systems*

I n the preceding two chapters we discussed the beliefs, assumptions, ideologies, and philosophies that are the basis of the human service model. In this chapter we will focus on the organizational patterns for the human services and deal with how the services are to be delivered. While it is important to have the proper philosophy, it is equally important to have an effective organization if services are to be delivered where they are needed. It is also important to keep in mind that there is no one correct organizational chart which will meet the needs of every situation. Even after an effective organization has been developed, there will still be changes, which will then create new problems. The organizational patterns must be fluid, sensitive, and adaptable. No human service organization should be static; instead, it should be in the process of ongoing and continuous change.

Organizations are created and grow in order to handle the

day-to-day functioning of human affairs. They provide an operational plan for transacting necessary business, whether the organization is a family or General Motors. Their primary function is to provide the ground rules for their daily operation, thereby, hopefully, eliminating confusion, duplication of efforts, and decisions made by the wrong people. This procedure should meet the needs of the group and never be an impediment. Unfortunately, in families as well as General Motors, once an operational procedure—good or bad—is established, it is difficult to change it.

Because of this difficulty of change (often called bureaucracy), organizations and their behavior have long been studied by citizens, politicians, and scientists. In this chapter, in presenting several organizational problems and issues that confront social service agencies, we will discuss the following issues:

- Why is it difficult for an organization to change its systems, procedures, and goals?
- How can an organization's manpower be helped in coping with and facilitating the necessary changes?
- How can we implement an effective strategy for communication and decision-making within an organization?
- What effects can be expected from changes designed to make the organization more adaptive and responsive to the present needs of its consumer group?

This approach to studying organizational patterns will highlight the necessarily transitional quality of "healthy" systems and the way in which they grow. Like individuals, organizations exhibit changes and developments that are adaptive and nonadaptive. Skills in organizational problem-solving can help avert the nonadaptive developments.

Problems and Processes of Organizational Change

Marshall McLuhan [1964] has said that we are living today in a "pop culture." Recent changes in the technology of electronic communication have not only made possible, but have forced, many changes in our lives. These changes, which we are expected to adjust to, are staggering. One has only to remember today's values, expectations, and products and compare them with those of 10 or even 5 years ago. Probably more changes have occurred and been adjusted to in the past 20 years than in all the rest of man's history. It would therefore seem logical that change within organizations would take place smoothly and consistently in order to meet new problems and demands; unfortunately this is not the case. Changes within organizations occur only with the greatest difficulty and are always accompanied by great acrimony and anguish. Resistance is an inevitable part of change.

Contrary to popular belief about the various mental health organizational systems, goals are not set and decisions are not reached through a logical, rational process. Rather, the day-to-day operation of most mental health establishments is managed much like medieval fiefdoms. The various services of an institution operate as a loose collection of formal and informal powers and influences under the direction of a chief administrator. Each service competes with the others for such things as more staff, nicer buildings, larger areas of responsibility, and more money for equipment and contractual services. The struggle is especially bitter, because there are rarely enough resources to go around. In order to get more, public relations campaigns attempt to convince the administrators higher up (as well as the public) that its programs provide more service with less staff than do comparable programs, and therefore have greater needs and should have higher priority for the available resources of the system. No one wants to give up anything. The service directors realize that there is a correlation between their piece of the pie and the size of their "turf": those with the most patients and largest staffs have the greatest need and thus the most influence and power. These struggles take place at all levels of the organization. They go on among hospitals, between programs within a hospital, between services within the same program, and even among staff members. This struggle has a very divisive and inhibiting effect upon the operation of the organization at every level.

Each organizational unit within a system simultaneously protects its "borders and frontiers" while raiding its neighbors—which, obviously, does not make for smooth and systematic change. In such systems, change occurs when the operations and priorities get so far out of line with the needs of the overall system that the disparity can no longer be tolerated and an organizational crisis occurs. The crisis produces wholesale changes, with entire programs being changed or

251

Institutions should meet the needs of a group and not be an impediment instead. Unfortunately, once a system—good or bad—is established, it is difficult to change it. United States Senator Jacob Javits witnesses a demonstration to improve Willowbrook. (Photo by Bill Stanton, courtesy Magnum.)

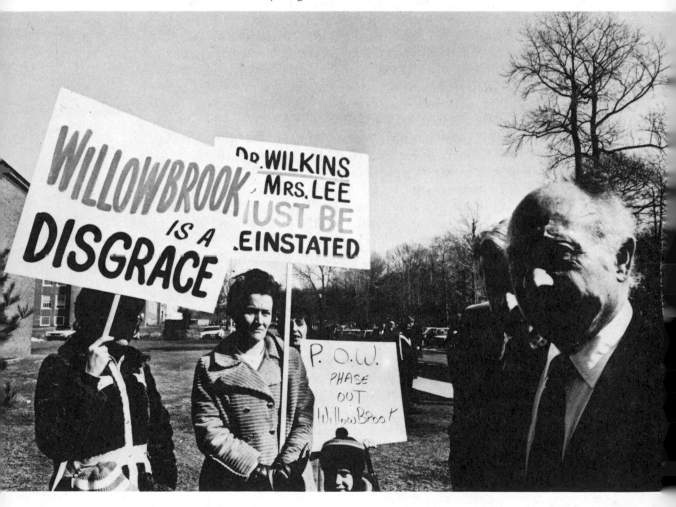

obliterated along with their resources. Building, manpower, and equipment are channeled into new operations and programs. The organizational crisis is similar to crises within an individual. Old values and priorities are exchanged for new ones. Old relationships between staff members are dissolved and replaced with new groupings. Lines of authority and communication change, and staff members attempt new job roles. Clearly, the extent and quality of the changes the staff and organizational system can and will tolerate far exceed the usual expectations. Following are two case histories of such changes, one at a large state hospital and the other at a community mental health clinic, which will help you understand the problems leading to change.

Institutional Conflict, Crises, and Reorganization

Agencies, like individuals, have great adaptive capacities. As long as an agency solves problems effectively, it will remain essentially stable and evolve in an orderly and meaningful fashion. It was the failure of this agency (the state hospital) to respond to pressures and needs in the 1940s and 50s that brought it to the point of crisis —approximately 7,000 patients, meager per diems, and no treatment beyond the intake wards. It was clear that something desperately needed to be done about the snake-pit situations confronting the institution. Changes had to be made which would lead to more effective use of existing resources, as it was clear that new resources—in the way of more staff, equipment, and new buildings—would not be forthcoming. Existing resources consisted largely of a custodial staff, a decaying physical plant, and an ineffective treatment technology. A feeling of desperation seems to have been the key ingredient in bringing about some pragmatic problem-solving, probably not only because of its motivational qualities, but because it tended to make apparent the real needs and priorities of the system. A great part of the agency's rejuvenation in the 1960s resulted from an increased sense of responsibility for the requirements of its patients, public, and employees. The agency has increased its skill in identifying needs and has developed greater skill in finding reasonable solutions to the issues confronting it:

Need: improved living conditions.

253

Approach: introduction of milieu therapy programs in 1961.

Need: greater flexibility to expedite change and increase innovations.
Approach: decentralization of the hospital into the unit system in 1963.

Need: increase patient-staff contacts regarding counseling, problem-solving, and planning.
Approach: beginning of the team approach in 1965, with staff being allocated to programs rather than to departments.

Need: provide wide range of services to maximum number of patients.
Approach: development of the generalist philosophy in 1965 and introduction of the career series, which has begun to peak only recently.

Need: accountability for patient service, attempt to give all patients "some of the action" (no option to decline), increased mental health service to the community.
Approach: development of catchment system in 1968.

Need: optimal use of personnel, elimination of poor physical plant and equipment, provision for increased services to infirmary and geriatric patients, and upgrading, standardization, and increase of services at admission point.
Approach: various reorganizations reflecting a change of the hospital status—(1) closing down of extended-care services and discontinuance of obsolete buildings; (2) uniting geriatrics and infirmaries; (3) establishing a new central admission service.

This approach—of identifying needs, problem-solving to meet needs, and the institutional reorganization that results from this process—is referred to as *Treatment Through Institutional Change* (Fisher, Mehr, and Truckenbrod [1973a and 1973b]). While in hindsight, all of these changes were for the improvement of the system's ability to respond to the various needs of its consumer group, at the time, the changes were considered so radical as to be dangerous, a conspiracy to destroy the hospital, and as unworkable and crazy.

Resistance consisted of passive-aggressive behavior, active sabotage, and at one point open rebellion when some of the staff marched on the superintendent's office. The reasons for the resistance were primarily the staff's fear of their possible incapacity to function competently in the new programs, their loss of turf and prestige, and their fear that they were going to lose their jobs and security. The changes brought great amounts of stress, which unfortunately probably led to a few people leaving the system and to some premature retirements.

The changes, however, led to more effective services for the agency's consumer group, as well as a staff that feels more effective and competent. Table 17.1 indicates that the changes have led to improved services. It demonstrates that as a result of the changes the hospital is now able to respond to more persons in trouble and then return them to the community.

Table 17.1

State Hospital Admissions Versus Total Population

Fiscal year	Total patients admitted	Total patient population
1961	2,595	5,850
1971	3,138	2,271

Crisis in a Community Mental Health Clinic

Our mental health clinic, which will be called the Downtown Mental Health Clinic, was organized under a federal grant to provide services to a large metropolitan community catchment area. The clinic was staffed by traditional professionals who were to provide counseling services to people in the community. Unfortunately, the agency director, as well as the staff, only saw "clients" in their office on a 9-to-5 basis. The clinic functioned for several years, with the staff seeing patients in their offices but doing little else. The members of the staff were not indigenous members of the community and, as a result, did not relate well to the residents and their special

255

problems. As time passed, the waiting list for services grew longer, since the staff preferred to work with those patients who were less trouble to work with.

The downtown area was a transitional neighborhood, going from bad to worse. As was symptomatic of the times (the mid- to late 1960s), street riots occurred in which buildings were destroyed by fire and looting. During one riot, the clinic was destroyed, along with businesses which, the local inhabitants felt, were run by outsiders who were no more than parasites on the neighborhood. These outsiders were store owners who drove into the neighborhood at 9 in the morning and out again at 5. They were obviously living off the neighborhood and not contributing anything to it.

The staff and agency director never returned to the neighborhood. There were, however, some unspent funds left in the account of the grant, and the federal government sent in an investigating team to determine what had happened, whether services were still required, and whether the clinic itself was valuable to the community.

From interviewing residents and local community leaders, the investigating team found out that the clinic had not provided the services the people needed, that the clinic staff could not relate to the indigenous problems of the community, that there was a vital need for relevant services, and that the local residents would make use of and support a clinic which could relate to their community and provide helping services. The remaining funds were turned over to community leaders who were to reopen the clinic and provide relevant services. These leaders formed an action committee to identify the resources and problems of the community. In its opinion, the community's primary need was not the traditional counseling services provided by the former clinic, but rather a set of brokerage services which would link the residents to existing resources. If none existed, the committee suggested contracting to have them developed and provided. This mode of operation was, of course, quite different, and it has been much more successful in the community, which sees it as its own program.

The important themes in organizational change are:

• There is no one ideal organizational chart for every human service agency.

• Changes in the problems and needs of the human services consumer group make changes in the organization of the services mandatory.

- Today's solutions are likely to be tomorrow's problems.

- It is difficult for an organization to continuously alter its operations and goals smoothly and consistently.

- The need for change usually has to reach the crisis stage before an institution will react with large-scale changes.

- When an institutional crisis occurs, staff of all levels react with fear, suspicion, resistance, and hostility. When staff are *in* a crisis, however, they are better able to adopt new attitudes, learn new skills, and participate in new programs.

- When an institutional crisis occurs, the institution has many resources for coping with the problems and demands. Important among these is the capacity to survey the problem, identify the need, and develop a pragmatic, problem-solving approach.

Helping Personnel Cope with and Facilitate Necessary Changes

When an agency is confronted with an organizational crisis and attempts to solve it, its staff members are under great stress and anxiety, which lead it to be fearful, suspicious, resistant, and hostile. This reaction usually consists of staff members not wanting to give up their existing relationships with other staff and patients, their job roles, and their work settings in exchange for strange, new tasks. This is a common reaction. The important question is not whether the change should occur, but how an organization's personnel can adjust to it. If the process is skillfully handled, the crisis and stress accompanying it provide an unusual opportunity to make major alterations in attitudes, skills, and job roles acceptable to the agency's staff. The management of changes in attitudes, skills, and job roles usually takes the form of new training. It is important that the training not be a random collection of vaguely related subjects. Training should focus on what the new job is about; the staff should be shown that it will help them survive in their new job assignments. For example, if a group of staff are brought together to work with chronic, withdrawn patients, the focus of the program development training might be behavior modification, token economies, level systems, or reinforcement therapy. Ideally, this training occurs in a problem-solving milieu where staff participate as a group working as a team, following the Program Development Project (Truckenbrod and Kostur [1972] see Appendix). Such an approach is a powerful alternative to traditional training, which in the past has approached training with classrooms, blackboards, *teachers,* and *students.* This method, which has been unable to involve the participants, must be reexamined. It is all too apparent that there are only a few charismatic individuals who are effective in delivering the training in a classroom situation. The classroom must be largely abandoned in favor of new training procedures. Ideally, these procedures should have the following objectives.

- They must increase the participation of all persons involved in the process.
- They must abandon caste concepts such as "student," "trainee," "teacher," "lecturer," and replace them with expectations that everyone involved in the learning experience has a *contribution* to make.
- They must study at a site in which actual, ongoing problems and processes are encountered and dealt with.
- The training experience should invest all members of a treatment team simultaneously. This strategy helps to counter problems arising when one or two employees are trained and then return to the ward, where their enthusiasm is diluted by the inertia of the existing program. With these objectives in mind, it seems clear that the organization's training efforts must be focused on the treatment team working as a group and delivering services to their target population within the framework of the treatment team's priorities and objectives. It is the treatment team, for example, that provides a behavior-modification program to a group of patients, crisis intervention services to residents of a particular community, or a physical rehabilitation and placement program to a group of geriatric patients. The effectiveness of such a treatment team depends on: clearly identified objectives; organizational qualities to work toward operationalizing their objectives; program knowledge and skills gained through consultation, informational discussion, and reading, which allow all members of a team to function competently; and evaluation and feedback systems to provide the team with in-

formation about the degree to which they are achieving their objectives.

It is in such a process as this that training will be most readily accepted and best utilized. If the treatment team is charged with providing mental health services to a community, the greatest needs the team will feel will be for information and consultation on the issues of developing an effective community organization, crisis intervention, aftercare, and developing working relationships with other community service agencies. If the treatment team is responsible for the rehabilitation of long-term institutionalized patients, they might be most interested in developing a behavior-modification program with a token economy, daily living schedules, and discharge planning. The need for specific kinds of training, organizational planning, and consultation comes from the service demands of the treatment team, and not vice versa. Following is an example of how this approach to training might operate.

The Design of Reception Service Training for an Admission Program

This team would be responsible for handling persons seeking admission to the agency from a community area surrounding the agency and for linking these persons either to the agency's outpatient service, to other community resources, or to short-term, inpatient treatment services.

The team might decide that they would like to have their program consist of a system of crisis intervention and thus link patients to a network of community services. In developing their new reception service, the team would:

• Begin to identify programmatic objectives, including: the prevention of inpatient hospitalization by crisis counseling in the community; linking potential patients to other community service agencies; developing skills in assessing patients' problems, social resources, and alternatives to and matching them with inpatient treatment; and developing crisis-intervention and problem-solving skills that would preclude extended hospitalization.

259

- Identify and recruit a consultant who has knowledge and skills pertinent to the program's needs.
- Attempt to build into regular team meetings opportunities for organizational development and realization of objectives.
- Find workshops and pertinent college-level training.
- Develop evaluation and information systems.

Such a method of training would help the staff cope with the problems of moving into new jobs, accepting new values, and learning new skills. In providing the staff with support and help, the training can channel the tensions and anxiety into useful and productive avenues. By participating in such program development projects, staff members may show unusual investment and commitment because they have not only been trained in the necessary skills, they have taken part in the design and implementation of the treatment program.

Implementing an Effective Strategy for Communication and Decision-Making

If an organization is to pursue its objectives effectively, it is crucially important that it work out a strategy for communication and decision-making. This means that within the organization certain decisions should be made at one level while others are made at another, all the while maintaining an appropriate level of information flowing between the various decision-making points to maintain the integrity of the entire system. This type of operation may be thought of as roughly analogous to a man walking to the store for a loaf of bread. If you consider the process of purchasing the bread as a collection of behaviors and missions, the analogy that follows becomes clear:

Operation	Level of Decision	System Feedback
1. Walking to the store	Spinal column, medulla, and musculature	Information about the walking procedure is generally kept at or below the level of consciousness unless it is interrupted. For example, the person encounters a newly poured concrete sidewalk.

2. Selecting the bread	Cerebrum	Information is recalled about the various qualities of the available brands and a decision is made. While the choice is usually consciously made, a great deal of involved planning and decision-making is usually not involved.
3. Purchasing the bread	Cerebrum	Here a complicated operation is involved. The buyer compares the price of the bread with previous prices. He then calculates the sales tax and compares the total purchase price with the amount requested by the sales clerk. If all of these decisions check out as being within the normal limits of the amount the buyer expects to pay, he completes the transaction.

In this example involving a routine function, the operation of an integrated, total system is seen as being comprised of various subsystems, each of which has a different responsibility. Decisions and general control are made at various points in the system. The necessity for efficiently managing the decision-making and internal communication (*feedback*) is immediately apparent. If the person in our example had to decide or be consciously aware of and in control of *every* step, he probably would have starved to death before he got to the store.

An example of such inefficient decision-making and communication on an institutional level is given in Part II as being part of the conditions that lead to a critical mass situation. There the decision-making procedure for discharging a patient from a service agency is involved. A nervous agency director reviewed every discharge in his office. At this level of the system's operation, decision-making regarding discharge was as inappropriate and cumbersome as the man who made a conscious decision about every step he took on the way to the store. The director's decision-making was inappropriate for the following reasons:

- Persons elsewhere in the system (closer to the patient) had more pertinent information based on day-to-day experience.
- The director could not hope to adequately familiarize himself with every aspect of every case which needed discharge action.
- The director did not have adequate time, even if this were his only function.
- If the director were making these kinds of decisions, other impor-

261

tant decisions he should have been making went by unattended—for example, the lack of programs in the hospital.

• Because of the director's visibility to the legislature, newspapers, and hostile relatives, he received the negative reactions from every discharge that failed. (People rarely give positive feedback about discharges that work out well.) This negative reinforcement quickly made him very cautious and unwilling to take risks in discharging patients, even those with a reasonably good chance of surviving in the community.

• Because the director was making all of the decisions about who got discharged and under what circumstances, the hospital staff working with the patient rarely got any experience or feed back in what kind of patient had a reasonably good chance to reenter the community successfully. Roughly speaking, skill in deciding who is a good prospect for discharge grows out of firsthand experience, in much the same way that basketball players learn to shoot free throws—not by watching someone else do it but by participating in the process, by making the decision, and then by watching what happens (feedback). This is the only way to become efficient in such areas.

The preceding examples both illustrate important principles of designing effective communication and decision-making within an organization:

• Regular operational decisions should be made at the level of the organization where there is the greatest amount of information. For example, the decision to discharge a resident should be made by a team or group of people who work daily with the resident, not by the director.

• Decisions affecting the priorities and resources of the organization as a whole should be made by the director or person ultimately responsible for the organization. In making decisions, the director should seek to distribute the organization's resources equitably. For example, he should make sure that all of the agency's programs have a roughly equivalent staff-to-patient ratio.

• Communication between all levels of the organization is essential. It must operate in all directions, both horizontally between programs and vertically between different levels of the organization.

The feedback between the subsystems of the organization communicates the needs of the treatment personnel (treatment teams), as well as the need for changes in operations and priorities. For example, the management policy of the organization might be to place all geriatric patients in private nursing homes rather than maintain a large inpatient population. Reasons for this might include (1) the belief that the geriatric patient will get better care in a private nursing home; (2) it is cheaper to place patients in new, privately-operated nursing homes than to upgrade the deteriorating physical plant of the state hospital; and (3) this policy conforms to the general practice of providing care for all mental health casualties within their own communities.

These reasons must be communicated and discussed with the staff responsible for putting the organization's policies into practice. In turn, the treatment teams who are called on to deliver the services must communicate their needs to management. These might include:

• The time and funds to develop programs designed to get all members of the treatment team on board with the total mission of placing the patients in private nursing homes.
• They may need some funds for giving patients rehabilitation in daily living skills, so they can survive when they are placed in a private nursing home.
• They may need transportation for delivering patients to nursing homes and office equipment for processing paperwork.

In addition to the communication of needs and policy, a third type of communication is needed to maintain the coordination between the treatment team and management. This type of communication should consist of daily feedback regarding the achievement of the goals and policies. The feedback should include information about the following:

• Patient movement—admissions, discharges, average daily census, readmissions
• Behavioral Rating Scales regarding general patient progress.
• Regular meetings between management and treatment teams to

263

keep abreast of changes, problems, needs—in short, the general progress of the program.

This system, which includes policy statements, communication of program needs, and regular feedback sessions, provides an effective, efficient, ongoing transfer of information which will insure an organization of at least some success in achieving its objectives.

In designing an effective decision-making strategy for an organization, care should be given to insure (1) that the decisions are made at the point where there is the greatest amount of information, and (2) that the agency director makes decisions designed to distribute the agency's resources among its various programs equitably. Patterns of communication should also be established within the organization, which will provide adequate information for coordinating policy and operations within the framework of program needs and the feedback of results. Effective decision-making and communication are vital to the delivery of services and the integrity and solidarity of the total organization.

Organizational Changes

The effects that can be expected from changes designed to make the organization more adaptive and responsive to the present needs of the consumer group may be categorized under two headings: positive effects within the organization and positive effects on the relationship between the organization and the public.

Internal Effects

The positive effects within an organization, from the viewpoint of adapting to the needs of the consumer, are primarily those of general staff attitudes and specific program effectiveness. The attitudes of the staff toward their working environment and roles depend on their feelings about the following:

Their feelings of involvement in the design and direction of the program with which they are involved. For example, if a human service worker feels that a socialization group involving window-shopping trips into the community would be effective, does anyone endorse and support this? If the worker feels he is being supported, that his suggestion was given a fair hearing, he will be encouraged to make suggestions and actively participate in the future. His involvement is vitally important in getting services to the patient.

Their feeling that the mission of the organization is essentially right and is contributing to, rather than detracting from, the consumer and his community. This means that the organization has no "Catch 22's" and that the community served by the organization value the organization and think of it as a responsible part of the community, whether it is a state hospital, community hospital, community mental health clinic, or some other specialized social service agency.

The positive effects of adaptive change and organization at the programmatic level consist of getting appropriate services to the consumer, based on what he needs rather than what the staff members would like to do. Positive effects of this type are characterized by: shorter periods of hospitalization; the reduced effect of institutionalization (which tends to be dehumanizing); greater frequency of contact including members of the patient's community, employer, family, friends, and other agencies; prevention of hospitalization by referring the patient to a functional network of community-based services and resources; and if hospitalization occurs, effective discharge planning and follow-up services designed to support the patient's reentry into the community.

External Effects

The positive effects on the relationship between the organization and its public are characterized by the following: adequate funding and financial support, support from other human service agencies based within the community, and support from the consumers and their social network. An agency's reputation for providing effective services is critically important to its existence in terms of receiving adequate funding from a legislature or tax board. This support determines the available resources of the organization, be it social service agency, community mental health clinic, or state hospital. This is especially true in today's economy where the staggering inflation diminishes the purchasing power of each tax dollar. A governing body is likely to reduce an organization's funding, especially when the organization has little support from its constituency. When the governor of a state prepares his budget, in which mental health must compete for funding with road-building and education, the size and support of the mental health constituency is all-important. The constituency—taxpayer-voter-citizens—can be rallied to support larger mental health budgets or to prevent cuts only if they feel they are getting some services they don't want cut because of inadequate funding in the state budget. It is at budget time that the support of the other human service agencies, as well as that of the consumer and his social network, becomes vitally important. It is imperative that the human service worker and his agency keep this in mind. The mandate for mental health funding is increasingly dependent upon an active and growing consumerism.

Summary

In this chapter we have related the philosophy and beliefs of the human service model to the implementing of effective organization patterns. It has been stressed that there is no one correct organizational chart that will meet the needs of every situation. Rather, organizations, like individuals, must grow by coping with and adapting to needs and problems. In this chapter the emphasis has been on the belief that organizational structure and strategy must grow out of the needs of the consumer rather than the wishes of staff members. In this way the human services will not only be able to provide pragmatic, problem-solving programs, they will be able to gain the support of the new consumer constituency.

Chapter 18 Delivery Systems and Technologies for the Human Services

*I*n this chapter we will see how services are delivered in the human service model, as well as the types of services, treatments, and technologies used by human service workers. In preceding chapters we have looked at the development of the human service model, its underlying beliefs and philosophy, and its organization. Here we will develop these into a perspective at the level of the delivery system, for example, public education, community mental health, behavior modification, integrity groups, and community organization. The basic difference between a delivery system and a technology is their level of application. For our purposes here, a *delivery system* will be considered as a general strategy for bringing services to consumer groups, such as a comprehensive community mental health clinic or a hospital. A *technology* is a specific plan or operation for effecting a change in an individual or group, such as behavior modification, group therapy, or crisis intervention. You should keep in mind that the technology, whatever it may be, is given shape and form by the delivery system in which it exists.

The primary objective of the human service model is the maintenance and support of the patient (or "client" or "consumer") in his own community. What this means for the individual human service consumer is that he should be able to maintain interpersonal transactions within his life space, that is, meet the requirements for living in his society. These transactions involve systems in the individual for the following purposes:

1. The intake of food, water, and information.
2. Establishing intimate, ongoing relationships.
3. Establishing relationships with a peer group.
4. Establishing a job role, an occupation or career.
5. Establishing a stable link with the cash economy.
6. Enabling a cherishable sense of self to be established.
7. Including a comprehensive system of meaning for the individual.

The maintenance and support of the individual and his systems, on both a day-to-day basis and during periods of crisis, occurs at three basic levels—prevention, crisis intervention, and rehabilitation. In this chapter we will discuss these three levels, but first we will provide a framework within which you should be able to organize the detailed information you will encounter in future training. Then we will provide a brief, detailed description of several innovative techniques and strategies.

The Orientation of the Delivery Systems

The delivery systems and technology of the human services occur at three stages of consumer need—*prevention*, the attempt to avoid crisis (maintain coping behavior and problem-solving); *crisis intervention*, in case the normal coping behavior is interrupted; and *rehabilitation* of the individual's coping systems, should they prove inadequate to sustain him in regular community life

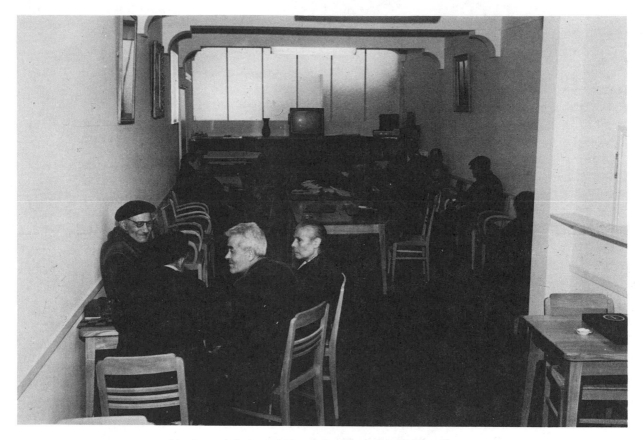

Neglect of the aged is a major human problem all over the world. Above: a meeting place for elderly Spanish refugees who otherwise would be isolated. (Courtesy Spanish Refugee Aid.)

Prevention

Prevention—in the breakdown of the coping behavior of the individual—is the preferred stage at which to plan for and deal with the human service needs and problems of the individual consumer, for the following reasons:

1. It reduces the risk of institutionalization and the dehumanization that can occur during the later stages of delivery services, during which the individual is without resources and thus more dependent. It allows him to maintain his position within his network of resources.

2. Prevention is generally less complicated and is more open to public scrutiny and evaluation. At this stage, the potential human service consumer can choose between alternate courses of action. Those that are most to the point and pragmatically solve the problem are the courses of action which will most often be subscribed to and supported.

3. Because the consumer makes use of relatively uncomplicated services and can bring his own resources into use, the cost to him and to the taxpayer is generally less. For example, if a community has inadequate recreational programs and resources for its youth, it is usually cheaper, as well as less risky and complicated, to spend tax money on a youth service center than on a youth correctional facility.

The problem with delivering services to an individual or community at the prevention stage is largely one of mobilizing and organizing the community when problems and dangers are still potential ones and not yet real ones. It is difficult to get community leaders and volunteers to take potential problems seriously and it is extremely difficult to prove that prevention systems have an impact on reducing deviance. The data on community deviancy is inadequate, which makes it difficult to establish that significant changes will result from prevention measures. Most communities are reactive, in that they tend to do nothing about their problems until something goes wrong; therefore there is minimal planning for human service systems.

A partial list of the human service activities and operations which could function at the prevention stage for a community are:

1. Educational programs for adults, as well as children and adolescents.
2. Family planning and abortion counseling services.
3. Individual and group health and accident insurance programs.
4. Occupational security for all members of a community.
5. Financial planning and counseling services at banks and other lending institutions.
6. Access to recreational facilities that are adequate for meeting the special needs and interests of all groups and ages in a community.
7. Counseling services for all age groups.
8. Children's day-care centers and well-baby clinics.
9. Youth programs.
10. Comprehensive community organizations.
11. Public safety including police, fire, and environmental protection.

These services must be accessible to all members of a community. Accompanying them must be an active and aggressive public education campaign which will make the citizens of a community aware of the programs and options available to them and encourage them to make use of the programs before situations and problems become crises. Analogous to preventive community programs are the semiannual trash removal services which some cities conduct, during which any amount of rubbish or unwanted materials is removed. This service helps prevent home fires, accidents, neighborhood decay, and disease and in so doing may save more homes from fire than does the local fire department. For much the same reason, people must organize and develop preventive human services. Just as it is simpler, more economical, and more humane to prevent fires than to put them out, it is simpler, more economical, and more humane to prevent human crisis than to provide crisis intervention services. To draw the analogy to its logial conclusion, communities should have a Human Crisis Prevention Week, with speeches by leading citizens, the opening of new human service projects, and

271

programs in the grade schools and high schools, complete with badges and hats. This is the only approach which will make the point to the public that it really is all right to take advantage of counseling and educational problem-solving programs before a real human crisis occurs. Prevention services need not be delivered in a brown paper bag.

RICHARD CORY*

Whenever Richard Cory went down town,
We people on the pavement looked at him:
He was a gentleman from sole to crown,
Clean favored, and imperially slim.

And he was always quietly arrayed,
And he was always human when he talked;
But still he fluttered pulses when he said,
"Good morning," and he glittered when he walked.

And he was rich—yes, richer than a king—
And admirably schooled in every grace:
In fine, we thought that he was everything
To make us wish that we were in his place.

So on we worked and waited for the light,
And went without the meat, and cursed the bread;
And Richard Cory, one calm summer night,
Went home and put a bullet through his head.

Richard Cory needed Human Services. It is not always possible to identify those persons in need. Citizens need to feel that it is as appropriate to seek human services as dental services.

Crisis Intervention

Just as it is not possible to prevent *all* fires, even with an adequate fire department, it is not possible to prevent *all* human crises, even with various kinds of crisis-intervention services. However, effective prevention *can* reduce the number and severity of crises events in a community.

*From *Chief Modern Poets of England and America.* ed. Gerald D. Sanders and John H. Nelson, 3rd ed., New York: Macmillan, 1943.

Personal human crises are not only normal but should be expected at every level of society. These crises events, and the resulting situational stress reactions, usually accompany the loss, real or imagined, of something very important and significant in the normal, day-to-day functioning of the individual.

For example, we might expect a mother to experience a severe situational stress reaction after the death of her young child. (Because the child was important to the routine of the entire family, one can be sure that the family will also be deeply affected.) Her whole routine is disrupted by the loss, and she must develop new living patterns, now totally different without the child. To appreciate the degree of shock this loss entails, one must examine the situation carefully. The child represented many things to the mother —companion, job role, intimate relationship, basic stimulation, and an important extension of herself. To help the mother and her family through the crisis period (usually less than a month), there must be adequate and appropriate crisis intervention and support. In many families, adequate social relationships already exist among the family's relatives and friends and no further crisis intervention is needed. In today's mobile culture, though, many families do not have an adequate social network to provide the necessary support, and a formal, community-based, crisis-intervention system is necessary. Service at the crisis-intervention level should have the following characteristics:

1. Treatment must begin immediately upon the request of the individual, his family, or his friends.

2. Treatment should ideally take place within the person's own social milieu, where he is firmly linked to the people and transactions that existed before the crisis.

3. The human service worker should intervene in the life of the person in crisis to insure that the worker is obtaining the most accurate and constructive information available.

The encounter between the human service worker and the person in crisis (in addition to his social network) should be brief, supportive, and focused on the immediate aspects of the problem. Every attempt should be made to engage him in regular life activities. This approach will reduce the risk of institutionalization and disenfranchisement from the community.

273

A partial list of the resources and technology available to the crisis intervention process are:

1. Linking or relinking the person's systems and resulting transactions, which include family, friends, job, physical resources, information, financial ties, a cherishable idea of self, and a capacity to make both large and small decisions.
2. Counseling and problem-solving services to the person and his family.
3. Traveling teams of other human service workers.
4. An open operation, so as to use these potential resource people: police, teachers, ministers, neighbors, friends, family, employer, firemen, telephone operators, bank officers, lawyers, and public aid officials.

If appropriately managed, crisis intervention will prevent the troubled person from being isolated from his community, his existing social network, and his life space. The objective of crisis intervention is not only to keep the person in his community and prevent long-term hospitalization but to help him maintain his life style. If this does not occur, the crisis-intervention process has failed, because it will have left the person with an inadequate life style, as well as being more prone to involvement in future crises. If this happens consistently, the community will soon develop a "colony" of chronic recidivists and marginally adaptive individuals who will be difficult to provide services for, will tie up available resources (tax money), and will limit the available service to the larger community.

Rehabilitation and Direct Services (treatment for chronic deviance)

The third phase in the delivery of services involves the rehabilitation, direct services to, and treatment of the nonfunctional systems of the individual and their accompanying capacity for interacting with the various parts of his life. For example, this means that an individual who is without a job role will need rehabilitation services to bring the job role back to its proper level. These services might include a sheltered-workshop experience, development of good work habits (being on time and able to work eight hours), job counseling, inventory of occupational interests, trial job placement, and follow up. In addition, persons who require rehabilitation service are usually handicapped in more ways than one (not necessarily in the physical sense). In addition to these services, our hypothetical human service consumer would probably require rehabilitation services in the areas of daily living, personal care, and various group experiences, which will enable him to better survive in the community when he attempts to become more independent. Rehabilitation is obviously the most complex and expensive stage at which to provide service to the individual; it is much easier and less complicated to deal with the person at either the prevention or crisis-intervention stages of service. In the rehabilitation stage, the person is often without resources and is entrenched in an interaction network of dependency, disinterest, and few skills. The best example of this is the long-term chronic patient in a state hospital or a sheltered-care facility. In many cases these facilities have become a human garbage dump where the unwanted and inadequate people of American society are discarded. Following is a case history of such a discard, a person who was disenfranchised from society, who accepted the standards of behavior of a back ward chronic patient, and who was subsequently rehabilitated.

A Case History in Rehabilitation

"Fred," the subject of this history, was first encountered by one of the authors as an inhabitant of a back ward filled with regressed, untidy, acting-out male patients. Fred was an unlikely candidate for rehabilitation. His hospital file showed a grim story of nearly lifelong incarceration in institutions and hospitals. His "career" began when as a child of 9 he began having trouble concentrating in the third grade following the death of his father and was placed in a state training school for the retarded.

The admission note at the state school described a quiet, slightly withdrawn boy with little in the way of disturbed behavior. A few years later Fred's problems and disablties were much more evident and severe. He was now diagnosed as severely retarded and being epileptic. In addition, it was reported that he was frequently untidy.

The state school was the milieu in which Fred was raised. He adjusted to an environment depleted of informational stimulation.

His intimate relationship, if any, were with other inmates or the custodial staff. His peer group was the other unfortunates with whom he was herded together. His "job role," or "career," was that of a disturbed, retarded, untidy epileptic. He had no ties to the cash economy, no sense of cherishable self, no chance to make decisions. He was closer to being a vegetable than a human.

When Fred was 18 he was unceremoniously placed in the state hospital where another 20 years went by, punctuated by epileptic fits, harvesting state hospital vegetables, electroshock therapy, chemotherapy, disturbed behavior, and an overnight, abortive attempt at being a farmhand.

Following a periodic hospital reorganization, one of the authors was put in charge of Fred's ward. One of the attempts to re-motivate the patients was to involve them in daily living projects which included light housekeeping chores. Fred became involved in the chores and began to react positively to his job assignment and the reinforcements he received from the staff which included cigarettes and positive praise. As was typical in a state hospital, there was a shortage of employees, in this case, the dining room adjacent to the ward where the patients ate. Someone suggested that perhaps Fred could give them a hand in the dining room wiping off tables and washing trays.

The suggestion was followed, and Fred was placed in the dining room on a work assignment. He tried hard and was encouraged by the staff. Within a week he was behaving appropriately and his dressing habits had greatly improved. During the next several weeks he spent progressively longer periods in the dining room and out of the ward. He quickly substituted the dining room workers for his fellow patients as his peer group and became the most reliable worker there. Several months passed and one of the regular employees retired. Because the job was unattractive and low-paying, it would be difficult to find a replacement.

Fred was offered the job. He could live temporarily in the ward as a "guest" and then in the community once he had saved enough money to pay for room and board. The plan proceeded smoothly. Fred was hired, discharged from the hospital, and has survived outside the hospital in his job, while living as a responsible, taxpaying citizen in the community.

Today Fred is a responsible, 56-year-old state employee. The unfortunate aspect of this "happy ending" is that some 40 years of his life were wasted for lack of a workable alternative to hospitalization.

As this case history illustrates, the rehabilitation process is complicated, time-consuming (particularly for the client), and very expensive, if one considers the cost of operating a state hospital ward or sheltered workshop. It is, however, the stage at which we must work with many of the clients.

Basic Themes of the Human Service Model

Providing the appropriate technology, service, therapy, or rehabilitation within the human service model must be done from a problem-solving orientation. It must focus on the present and emphasize changing the client's environment rather than the inner man. The model can best be understood if each of the basic themes is examined.

Problem-Solving

This is essentially an assessment, or diagnostic service. The client arrives at the service agency for help. It is the task of the service-giver and the client to identify the problem, set a goal, and develop a method for solving the problem. Sometimes the problem is easily identified, the goal and method are clear because there are few options available. As an example, a client is broke, he has no friends or relatives he can borrow from. He is completely cut off from the cash economy. One answer is to link him to public aid (welfare).

On the other hand, the service-giver and the client may be able to find another solution. They might pursue the short-term goal of placing the client on the welfare roll while choosing a long-term goal to work toward. That is, they may plan for a more meaningful tie into the cash economy than the welfare system.

The service-giver and the client sit down and consider all possible solutions to the client's financial problem. They list the options:

Identify the client's chances of employment.
Discuss the possibility of training and/or futher education.

277

Discuss the job market and the sources of employment.

Discuss methods of seeking jobs.

Discuss how one should handle job interviews.

Discuss the client's need for inner change (therapy) before pursuing a job.

Identify jobs that are tied into a career series (see pg. 291).

Such a list should be developed uncritically and should include as many items as possible, regardless of how unrealistic they may seem at first. After the list is completed, the task is to go through the possibilities critically, reducing them to probabilities. Once this is done, the service-giver and the client examine the list in terms of the client's resources, capacities, interests, values, and age. This sets the stage for a decision. Once a decision has been made, the goal is set, which leaves the service-giver and the client the task of finding a method of achieving the goal.

Ten years ago one of the authors had a female client who was not content with her marriage. Although unhappy, most of her security and safety needs were being met, as were those of her five children. But her only tie with the cash economy was *through her husband* so a divorce was out of the question. The conflict was painful and difficult. At the time the client came in for treatment, she had not graduated from high school, nor did she have any work skills. The therapy was aimed at helping her develop a career and thus free her from economic dependency, so any subsequent decision would be based on her desire to remain married rather than on a feeling of financial dependency. During the next 10 years:

She was encouraged to take an examination for a high school degree (General Educational Developmental Test), which she passed.

She entered college.

She found a part-time job in an agency, which could lead to a career as well as pay for college.

She received—in turn—Associate of Arts, Bachelor of Arts, and Master of Arts degrees.

She obtained a position commensurate with her educational achievements and eventually surpassed her husband's salary.

She divorced her husband.

This is an example of the problem-solving orientation. It is at the core of all rehabilitation, or human service, therapies. The major task in serving a client is to get the problem-solving process going.

Here and Now

It has been customary in attempting to rehabilitate, treat, or service a client to examine him in great depth in order to find the cause of his problems. The human service model attempts to deal in terms of the here and now. The question is, what is occuring in the client's present that is causing his particular behavior? This is, of course, also part of the problem-solving process. In traditional therapies, there has been considerable emphasis on combing the individual's childhood trying to find out what happened in the family, what interactions there were that might have influenced the present deviance. These excursions into the past have resulted in therapy that can last five to ten years, if not indefinitely.

Altering the Environment

In the intraorganismic approach, when service-givers, therapists, or rehabilitation workers thought of helping the clients, they meant somehow *changing* him. It was assumed that if the individual could not solve his problems satisfactorily, there was something wrong with him, that the inner self must be altered. This leads to medication, lobotomy, psychotherapy, group therapy, or a combination of these.

On the other hand, the human service model assumes that the client's problems are frequently not so much *within* him as they are caused by social institutions. For example, it is implicit in our culture that there will always be some unemployment (around 3 to 5 percent). Many who happen to be among that 3 to 5 percent will go into a crisis because of being cut off from the cash economy, yet the cause of the problem is the economic system and not the individual. The task is not to treat this 3-5 percent with psychotherapy but rather to find a way to link the people in that statistical category to the cash economy. In addition, each society should continuously assess its social institutions and study their impact on its members.

For those individuals considered deviant, disturbed, or chronically failing to adapt, it is important to consider the possibility of altering, expanding, or creating new social institutions.

Following are some of the technologies for providing human services at the rehabilitation and therapeutic levels. These services will be discussed later in this chapter:

behavior modification
sheltered workshops
daily-living-skill training
spin-off groups
integrity groups
individual problem-solving
relinking operations
halfway houses
trips into the community
Synanon-type operations
aftercare

Rehabilitation and therapy can upgrade the behavior of most persons who do not have adequate resources to a point where they can survive in the regular community. It should be kept in mind that it is not only the people in state hospitals and sheltered-care facilities who need rehabilitative, therapeutic human services, but the many living in flophouses, fleabag hotels, on the street as alcoholics, and in the ghettos. The limit to who can be served is based on a community's resources. It is especially disquieting when one not only contemplates the cost of rehabilitation services for these people, but their cost as wasted resources, as Freds, when they could be contributing members to society instead of merely being liabilities.

Summary of the Human Service Delivery System

The first section of the chapter has dealt with the orientation of the human service system. Services are generally considered to be provided at three stages:

Prevention in the breakdown of normal coping behavior.

Crises intervention should the coping behavior be interrupted.

Rehabilitation programs to restore adequate coping behavior.

Table 18.1 summarizes the services.

Table 18.1
Delivery Systems and Technology of the Human Services

FUNCTION

Prevention	*Intervention*	*Rehabilitation*
The components of the person's system should provide an adequate set of transactions which will either prevent crises or reduce the possibility of the components being lost.	During a crisis, services are required which will help the person maintain his previously inadequate subsystem components.	When the components of the person's various subsystems are inadequate they must be replaced and restored.

TECHNOLOGY

Public education	Linking and relinking operations	Behavior modification
Family planning services	Counseling and problem-solving services	Workshops
	Traveling teams	Daily living skills
Group accident and health insurance	Resource groups	Spin-off groups
Occupational security	police	Integrity groups
Financial planning and counseling	teachers	Individual problem-solving
Adequate recreational facilities	neighbors	Relinking operations
Public safety services	friends	Halfway houses
Counseling services	family	Trips into the community
Youth programs	employer	Synanon-type operations
Comprehensive community organizations	firemen	Aftercare
	telephone operators	
	bank officers	
	lawyers	
	public aid officials	

Selected Human Service Therapies

In describing some human service therapies, we do not intend to suggest that these therapies are the sole province of the human services. All therapies, or technologies, regardless of the models that generated the therapies, can be used by a service-giver. Service-givers are primarily problem-solvers who become increasingly effective as the number of options (therapeutic techniques) available to them increase.

281

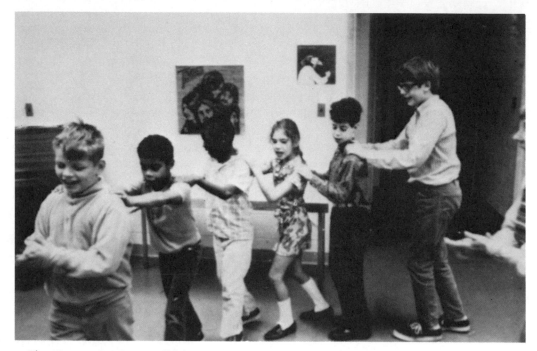

The Human Service model favors the maintenance of the patient in his own community. Below a local clinic for the young. (Photo by Costa Manos, courtesy Magnum.)

The sick child cannot easily become the well-adjusted adult. Here is a Holy Ghost father helping children in Biafra during the Nigerian-Biafran War. (Photo courtesy Holy Ghost Fathers and Father Aloysius Dempsey.)

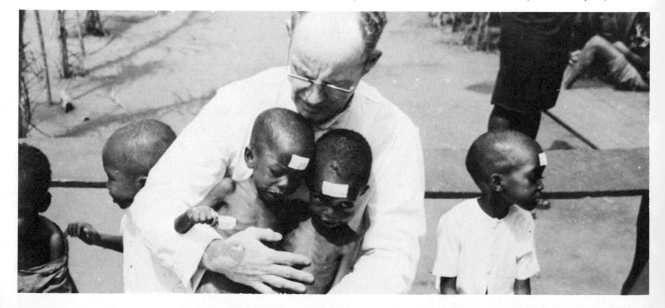

In many situations, other treatment alternatives are appropriate. The emphasis, of course, should be on the particular problem of the consumer, not on the technology per se. For example, we consider behavior modification an effective technology in many situations, but it is certainly not to be applied blindly every time a difficult problem occurs. Even if behavior modification *is* the appropriate therapy, it must be used intelligently. Technologies, whatever they might be or whoever uses them, must not be done automatically or by rote. Each person who seeks human services has unique circumstances and problems; it would be irresponsible for the human service worker to recommend or initiate a particular technology system without thoroughly understanding these circumstances and problems. Whenever possible, the human service worker should make every effort to involve the consumer in the selection and application of therapy as well as explain to him what the alternatives and possible consequences are. In addition, in cases where the consumer has a diminished ability to understand the alternatives and consequences of the therapy, the human service worker must assume an even greater level of responsibility and consideration. Examples of technologies being applied in wholesale fashion, and their sad consequences, unfortunately fill volumes of medical records. Here are some examples:

When lobotomies became popular, traveling teams of psychosurgeons went from hospital to hospital damaging the central nervous systems of patients, regardless of, and without any study of, the persons' problems and symptoms or of the side effects.

When sensitivity and encounter groups became a popular fad, everyone was encouraged to become more sensitive and to reach out and "touch their neighbor." While it is nice to be sensitive, indiscriminate use of the procedure has left many damaged and unglued people wandering the streets. Encounter groups are not for everyone.

When behavior modification became popular, many "helpers" felt they now not only had license to *reward* good behavior but to *punish* bad behavior. Unfortunately, many of them spent more time and energy punishing than rewarding.

The examples are virtually endless. It is therefore very important that therapy technologies be selected and implemented with the greatest of care and that the choice involve the consumer as often as possible. What seems expedient and effective at the time will be reviewed by future human service workers in the harsh light of the consequences of the particular technology.

We will now turn to several technologies in the human services. They fall roughly into the categories of prevention, intervention, and rehabilitation.

Technologies at the Prevention Level

Community organization is a recent type of applied social science which attempts to mobilize the existing resources of a community and to develop communication between the agencies, resources, and citizens. In this way the organizers hope to reduce stress and problems at the community level, which lead to emotional problems and crises on the individual level. Ideally, the organizers try to find solutions to problems before they occur. The focus of a community organization varies with the particular problems of the community. A typical pattern for suburban communities which have developed largely as residential areas is as follows:

First stage: young married couples buy new homes and have children.
Need: schools, fire protection, police departments, hospitals and mental health services.
Solution: organize support for and pass taxes to support institutions.

Second stage: many of the families have school-age children.
Need: parks, swimming pools, and other recreational facilities.
Solution: organize community park districts.

Third stage: many families have high-school-age children.
Need: adequate programs to occupy their time.
Solution: set up community-based youth programs, complete with recreational and counseling services.

Fourth stage: children leave families for college and jobs.
Need: for the first time in 20 years, parents have time on their hands and they are looking to the community for recreation.

284

Solution: set up an adult community organization, including reading groups, libraries, and garden clubs.

Fifth stage: adults retire from jobs.
Need: counseling and recreation services for senior citizens.
Solution: organize groups that will keep people involved and active. Help them understand their changed roles and how to relate to them. Set up counseling services for people as they lose spouses.

This simple example demonstrates the kinds of services citizens of a community might need over a period of years. These services become even more important when one considers the changing pattern of family life and the role of neighbors. Few people today stay in a community or even a section of the country long enough for "helpful home-town extended family" relationships to develop. Because the natural processes of community development require many years if not generations, community organizers are called on to help deliver the necessary service to the people and to prevent many human problems from reaching crisis proportions.

Technologies at the Crisis Intervention Level

Most crisis intervention centers are located where they are most accessible to the community, as well as being convenient to other human service agencies such as community-based drug programs, schools, rehabilitation centers, and public safety programs. There should be walk-in access in addition to telephone access. The crisis intervention center usually coordinates several operations which are designed to meet the needs of persons who are in trouble themselves or are interested parties.

The Screening-Linking-Planning Conference

The screening-linking-planning (SLP) conference is a meeting of the interested and significant people in a person's life, who together seek to help reorganize the person's coping behavior in crises (Hansell [1968]). People involved in such conferences, besides the person at the center of the crisis, may be members of the immediate family, friends, employer, minister, neighbors, police, and anyone else who expresses interest.

The SLP conference is a one-time event which sets the tone of subsequent interventions as they are needed. The meetings should focus on the temporary nature of the crisis and avoid becoming involved in a discussion of the person's behavior which may be disruptive, withdrawn, hostile, overly dependent, or suspicious. The emphasis should be on the pre-crisis functioning of the person and the post-crisis expectations. For example, if an SLP conference team works with a man who is exhibiting disruptive, confused, and suspicious behavior, they should attempt to assemble the various factions of his life space—wife, children, employer, neighbors, police, and clergy—using the following agenda:

1. An inventory of the person's life space (in terms of the seven basic transactional subsystems given in Chapter 15) is made. Transactions:
   (a) involving food, water, and information
   (b) on an intimate level with members of his family
   (c) on a peer group level with friends and neighbors
   (d) involving his job role and employer
   (e) with the cash economy—getting and spending money
   (f) involving his sense of self and of being worthwhile
   (g) involving the decision-making process—"this is better than that; I should do this first."
2. The group identifies the positive, pre-crisis characteristics and qualities of the person. For example, if the man in question has been a good provider and neighbor, the emphasis of the discussion should revolve around these issues. This usually leads the group to make positive associations to the person.
3. The person in crisis assumes a temporary time-out role, during which he is not accountable for most of his normal day-to-day responsibilities but instead, focuses his attention on reintegrating the normal transaction process, identifying the problem that led to the crisis, and attempting to problem-solve.
4. The expectation is established, for both the person in crisis and the group, that the time-out role is temporary and that the crisis is time-limited—24 hours to two weeks—and that following the crisis, the person will resume his pre-crisis level of functioning. (Most crises are episodic and will pass in time.)
5. Every attempt is made to confine the major treatment effort to

the person's own environment, because his family and friendship network has the greatest therapeutic potential. (This also makes it possible for the traveling team to get the best information about what is really going on.)

6. The person is linked to agencies *within the community* when specialized problem-solving services are required such as job counseling, financial support, or housing.

Conducting the crisis intervention in general and the SLP conference specifically with this agenda will maximize the person's problem-solving and coping abilities while minimizing the dangers of institutionalization and disenfranchisement.

Technologies at the Rehabilitation Level

The focus of the rehabilitation level technologies is on people who, while not in crisis, have difficulty coping independently, who have difficulty developing and maintaining such things as job, peer and intimate relationships, or decision making processes.

Behavior-modification is a broadly defined technology which uses principles from learning theory that have been developed in experimental laboratory situations, initially with rats and cats and later with human subjects. Behavior-modification technology is based primarily on the belief that behavioral responses that are rewarded tend to recur with greater frequency, while unrewarded (or punished) responses occur less often and eventually stop. The principle of reward and punishment has been elaborated on and added to over the last 30 years until at least a dozen theories have been developed by such men as Clark Hull [1943], K.W. Spence [1956], O.H. Mowrer [1960], and B.F. Skinner [1969]. In practice, however, most programs have relied exclusively on the alteration of behavior by manipulation of the positive reinforcement because of the dangers and the questionable ethic of using procedures that rely on negative or disagreeable conditions.

Most behavior-modification programs attempt to structure and motivate behavior which progressively approximates that of "normal," independently functioning, human beings. American society operates and is maintained largely through behavior-modification techniques applied unknowingly by either the party doing the reinforcing (rewarding) or the person being reinforced. For example,

287

most people are conditioned to go to work in the morning and home in the evening by a complex system of reinforcements involving paycheck, wife, children, home, and other factors. Patients who are long-term chronically institutionalized or socially disenfranchised are put on behavior-modification treatment programs. These programs attempt to upgrade the patients' level of functioning through behavior-modification and milieu-therapy programs.

A Behavior-Modification Program in a State Hospital

The objectives of these programs are remobilization and remotivation—for those patients who can attain it, the privilege of functioning outside the hospital; for those who cannot, increased self-esteem and comfort within a structured hospital setting. These programs apply a system of rewards in an effort to change behavior; they make the ward environment as much like the outside world as possible. Patients are rewarded for behaving in ways the community will accept. Since the patients' environment is controlled by the staff, the patient gradually learns, or relearns, behavior acceptable in that kind of environment.

A token economy provides the framework within which other activities take on increased importance. Patients are rewarded with tokens for appropriate behavior, which includes industrial therapy and on-ward assignments; participation in activities, program groups, ward meeting, etc.; and self-initiated activities or assignments. The tokens are redeemed for merchandise in the ward "store," such merchandise being toiletries and notions not otherwise available to the patients.

The activities and program groups are planned with the patients' needs and interests in mind. Each patient is encouraged to participate in the planning and to be involved as a member of a committee. Those unable to do this are encouraged to perform simple but necessary tasks essential to successful activity.

In including the patient in the program, this evaluation is done:

1. Determine what behavior needs to be changed.
2. Determine what is rewarding to the individual.
3. Settle on a plan of action, compiled from the knowledge learned in steps 1 and 2.

4. Carry out the plan consistently.

5. Observe the individual as the plan is carried out; evaluate and change it if necessary.

The goal of this program is to prepare the individual to cope with the demands of a less structured and more independent living situation which demands behavior appropriate to the outside community. The individual may have to develop habits of good dress, keep on a schedule, take care of personal belongings, and learn to react appropriately to normal expectations of the community. Additional examples of programs that use behavior-modification techniques are sheltered-care workshops and training programs for the mentally retarded.

As the rehabilitation theme is developed, it is important to understand that many different service-givers have designed and created a variety of technologies as solutions to a host of problems. There is nothing secretive or mysterious about the development of services; every parent is involved in the process just by working out his own family problems.

Integrity Groups

Integrity groups and therapy, which are examples of the small-group trend, have been initiated and promoted by O.H. Mowrer [1966] as a response to what he feels is the ineffectiveness of individual psychotherapy conducted by highly trained and paid professionals. Mowrer's views come from a lifetime of studying personal emotional problems and human turmoil. Over the years, he has rejected the deterministic theory in which man is a victim of his heredity and environment. He feels that every individual is responsible for his own decisions and for his own behavior. Each person has a conscience, or sense of right and wrong, which is the basis for his decisions. Mowrer feels that the individual runs into trouble when he violates his conscience or comprehensive system of meaning when making decisions and acting on them. For Mowrer, this kind of behavior leads the person to feel guilty and if not corrected, leads to various neurotic symptoms. Mowrer's formula for correcting these mental-illness-producing situations is for the person to become publicly accountable for the violations of his conscience rather than attempt to cover them up. In addition to being accountable, the person must make restitution that is appropriate to the acknowledged failure. Mowrer's formula includes a general responsibility for people to be open and honest in their relationships with each other.

This approach was first developed as a traditional therapy for helping persons crippled by an inability to relate to others. Since its origination, however, the approach has come to include the development of groups which meet regularly to discuss their relationships with other people, both inside and outside the group. Mowrer believes that these group-relationship experiences are vital to the regular routine of people, that they fill a vacuum caused by the frequent breakdown and failure of such institutions as the church and neighborhood.

Mowrer's concern about the breakdown of the traditional ability of institutions to link people to one another is reflected in a book by Fisher, Mehr, and Truckenbrod [1973]. They feel that institutions such as schools, churches, and families must be changed or new ones created, if people are going to be able to participate in vital growth experiences.

Modules of experience, which help a person grow, are the core of the rehabilitation concept. If, for example, a person has difficulty managing his finanacial resources and is thereby relegated to an ineffective and unhappy life style, he should have access to the modules of experience that will help him put his financial house back in order. The entire notion of rehabilitation modules is a basic theme of the human service model. The human service worker's focus in rehabilitation should be on identifying and implementing experiences that will help people grow, rather than using prepackaged systems that are not tailored to the needs of the person in trouble.

Many therapists working with clients with chronic maladaptive patterns have designed new therapeutic, or rehabilitative, programs, some of which are given below.

Spin-Off Groups

Rehabilitative workers such as George Fairweather [1964] have concluded that many long-term maladaptive persons are unable to live independently in the community. Fairweather's solution is to form cohesive groups of such persons, help them develop a business and appropriate living arrangements, and "spin them off" from the hospital as a group. This is a new pattern of living, in which personal resources of many people are combined.

Career Series

Many persons, when growing up, miss the opportunity for sufficient education, training, or preparation for a career, which results in their feeling alienated and detached from the mainstream of society. The *Career Series* represents a second chance. When an agency designs an effective career series, it provides the opportunity for someone to start at or near the bottom and through hard work reach the top. It's the theme that everyone can become President. The design for a Career Series is in a document by Mehr, Truckenbrod, and Fisher [1973].

Alternatives to Hospitalization

Most state hospitals were overwhelmingly crowded in the 1950s. A major factor in this overcrowding was the lack of alternatives to hospitalization. Starting in the mid-fifties and continuing up to the present, there have been a number of alternatives—quarterway houses, halfway houses, sheltered-care facilities, transitional care programs, day hospitals, and night hospitals. These are treatment alternatives between full time hospitalization and independent living.

In addition to these alternatives, a number of mental health care-givers who have rebelled against the medical model and the traditional service system have proposed and even designed new residential systems. R.J. Laing [1969] and Benjamin and Dorothea Braginsky [1973] suggest that those persons who have been locked up in residential facilities are not sick, just different. Their suggestions included the concept of new "asylums" which recognize and tolerate differences and are managed by the residents.

There are probably as many technologies to aid in the process of rehabilitation as there are life solutions to life's problems. It becomes the task of the human service worker to identify and authenticate those human experiences that will help a person grow and increase his skill in coping and problem-solving. The worker should

291

concentrate on the problem-solving process, not the technology, of human services.

Summary

In this chapter we have dealt with delivery systems and technologies for the human services. These helping services are provided at three stages of consumer need—prevention, intervention, and rehabilitation. There is more economy in providing services at the prevention stage than at the intervention or rehabilitation stages, because to do so is cheaper, less complicated, less dehumanizing and institutionalizing. You should also keep in mind the advantages of successful intervention as opposed to the rehabilitation strategy, because (1) it is also cheaper and less complicated, (2) it is very short-term, requiring few staff hours, and (3) it prevents the individual from becoming dehumanized and institutionalized.

In this chapter we also discussed the importance of involving the consumer in the choice of a technology, as well as the responsibility of the human service worker when initiating a treatment plan. Without these considerations, there is a tendency to fall back on the cliche, "the doctor knows best."

Chapter 19 *The Human Service Professions–Their Role, Function, and Training*

*T*he human service professions: roles, functions, and training have been emerging phenomena in the last ten years. They have grown out of the problems generated by a system based on specialized, segmented departments. These departments such as psychiatry, psychology, social work, and nursing, established roles which were both separate and arbitrary with regard to what services were to be provided to the consumer. Large amounts of time and energy were expended in warring over the definition of roles for each profession. Untold years have been wasted, for example, in attempting to prescribe what the proper role of the psychologist was to be and developing a technology to go with it. The most unfortunate result of this kind of role building activity was that it clearly did not serve the needs of the consumer. Rather than helping the consumer "put it back together," the division of labor tended to further split and divide the resources of the patient.

Out of these kinds of problems and resulting disintegration of service new solutions began to emerge:

The human service worker must be more than the sum of the various specialties. Training him does not mean teaching him a little psychology, a little social work, and a little psychiatry. It is a new configuration or gestalt of activities.

In treating a patient in the past, mental health specialists concentrated on an interpersonal relationship, verbal communication, and highly differentiated therapies having to do with the "mind." The human service worker today should be able to work with people in all walks of life. He must be willing to do whatever is necessary to help the patient. As a generalist, he must function as treater, advocate, and expediter.

The best analogy to the role of the human service worker is the home and the parents, for there the parents must participate in a variety of roles in order to facilitate the development and growth of their children.

In the past 10 years mental health care-givers have begun to reconsider the primary therapy systems. Treatment is more than using specific therapies such as chemotherapy, individual psychotherapy, or group therapy. It has become more closely linked to the activities in the "other 23 hours" of the day—the daily routines of life, the patient's relationship to a cash economy, the patient's occupational development. These latter concerns are part of the human service worker's role.

Philosophy of the Human Service Worker

Here are some ideas that express the philosophy of the human service worker:

It is better to provide some treatment for everybody rather than a lot of treatment for some and no treatment for others.

A treatment staff is required to do a little bit of everything (a bowling team), rather than being superspecialists on certain intervention techniques (a baseball team).

With few exceptions, everybody does everything—the work load is divided into equal units with an equal distribution of labor.

Treatment is available at all times of the day or night, rather than at specific times.

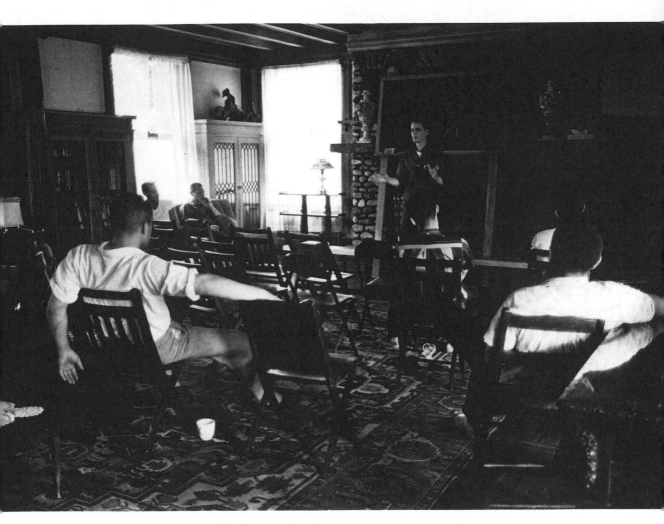

Human service in which the worker acts as treater,
advocate, and expediter. Here, a Synanon meeting.
(Photo by Charles Harbutt, courtesy Magnum.)

Class and caste differences between staff members and patients are minimized.

Staff Reaction

When staff personnel first encountered this philosophy, they were apprehensive and even hostile. This reaction came not only from social workers and psychologists but from psychiatric aides. To the professional staff, helping patients with everyday tasks was "beneath" them. The idea that it was "all right" for a psychologist to mop a floor and to help shower infirm patients was met with shock and disbelief. One muttered, "My mother didn't raise me to mop floors." For him, it was not a question of whether a floor needed mopping or that a patient might need help getting dressed; it was, "How can they expect this of *me*?" Staff professionals really believed that there was a class and caste difference between themselves and the aides (who traditionally did the lesser, menial tasks) and that they really were "too good" to be expected to meet the baser needs of the patients.

The problem of job expectancy was also shared by the psychiatric aides, who were now expected to participate in groups, fill out forms, help develop and implement treatment programs, and so on. They were afraid their jobs were going to be taken over by others, and as a result, either became passive-aggressive or started writing anonymous letters to the state legislature with hints that the patients were not receiving adequate care.

Activities the Human Service Worker Performs

The new employees, because they had few built-in expectations about what they would or would not be doing, moved into their new human service jobs and training with ease. Here is a partial list of the activities the new human service worker performs, regardless of educational achievement:

1. All treatment staff work on all shifts at one time or another, including weekends. In this way, service to patients is extended beyond the usual Monday to Friday, 8 A.M. to 4 P.M. shift to include

evenings and weekends, which allows more of the staff to participate in those important off-hour activities such as recreational programs and visits of relatives.

2. All treatment staff participate in all operations of the treatment program, which helps put activities in perspective. For example, if part of a treatment program is to develop daily living skills, a supervised program of dusting, making beds, and mopping floors is called for. Supervising patients in these activities was usually seen as a necessary but unimportant chore best done by the aide or attendant. This kind of thinking, however, misses the point of the important therapeutic quality inherent in these daily activities. Very often patients fail to survive when discharged into the community because of inadequate daily living skills.

3. All staff are expected to help maintain program accountability through the use of routine forms and patient evaluation. This usually takes the form of various team members, aides, human service workers, social workers, psychologists, or nurses, each acting as "counselors" for a number of patients. It involves progress notes, periodic reviews, program evaluations, discharge paperwork, requests for money, and home visits.

4. All staff are expected to participate in all specialized activities that involve the patients, such as conducting interviews, dispensing medication, and running the various kinds of group therapy. This helps maintain a team feeling in which the staff do most of the routine jobs, and so avoids the risk of certain groups monopolizing specialized tasks.

5. All staff are expected to participate in training events designed to improve the level of program functioning. This involves providing the entire team with a set of treatment skills they can use in their program. Such training avoids having one or two team members go outside the hospital to attend classes, workshops, or seminars and then return to the program hoping to involve other team members in their new experience, only to have their hopes crushed by the daily press of business.

6. All staff members have a right to expect a *workable* career ladder in which they may be rewarded for their training, energy, and responsibility rather than by their academic degree. *Job competence* is to be rewarded, not academic achievement.

As a general rule, specific staff activities in human services vary more between programs than within programs. In the traditional medical model, if you know what a social worker is doing in one program, you can fairly accurately predict what other social workers in other wards are doing. However, in the human service style of operation, the particular duties of staff vary greatly from program to program but little within one program.

There are no specific job roles that necessarily apply to all human service workers in all facilities, in that a particular individual's responsibilities are defined largely by the needs of the patients. Human service jobs, therefore, can be described only in specific situations. The following case study describes a human service at a residential children's treatment center.

JOB ROLE OF A HOUSEPARENT

A. To see to the physical, mental, and emotional needs of each child on an individual basis.

B. To have a houseparent available to the child on a 24-hour basis. It is important that the child knows that there is someone available (even during the night).

C. The houseparent accompanies the child on outings, whereas normally a mother or father would see to such shopping trips, where the child needs help in selecting the right clothing.

D. The houseparent counsels the child and listens to his problems and suggests alternative solutions.

E. It is up to the houseparent to see that each child lives up to his responsibilities:

    1. Keeping his room neat, performing his duties (such as clearing the table).

    2. That each child keeps dorm and house rules and if they are broken that the appropriate discipline is provided (such as being confined to the dorm or missing a special activity).

F. It is up to the houseparent to see that the child learns things he would normally have learned at home such as:

    1. table manners

    2. hygiene (baths, brushing teeth, etc.)

    3. proper grooming and dress.

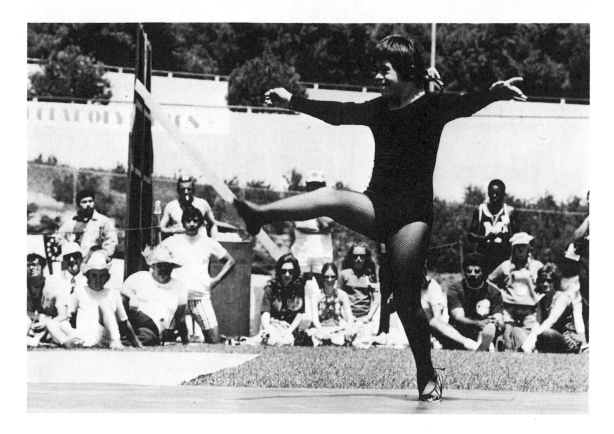

Examples of the function of the human service worker, the organization and fulfillment of the "special olympics" for the mentally retarded. (Helen Brush photography, courtesy The Joseph P. Kennedy Jr. Foundation)

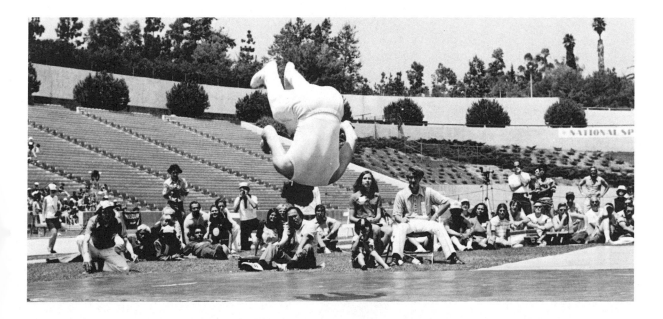

G. The houseparent must see to it that the child takes his proper medication, that a doctor is called if the child becomes ill, and that he has regular check-ups.

H. The houseparent must cooperate with the rest of the staff in
  1. Providing for the child's welfare.
  2. Seeing that the child follows his planned "treatment."
  3. Giving regular reports on the child's behavior and progress.

[Dianne Danielson]

Human Service Job Roles

Since every human service worker participates in a new, unfolding role, it should help to define what the human service professions are intended to be. While the human service worker is increasingly finding expanding job roles and opportunities across the country, these new roles are not eagerly accepted in all states. It will probably take at least 10 years for most states to develop personnel slots and job descriptions to accommodate human service workers. Indeed, it may be necessary for the new human service worker to enter the system in a traditional job such as "social worker trainee," "psychology intern," or "psychiatric aide." The title doesn't matter at this point. What is important is that the human service worker, operating under a pseudonym, goes to work in his job. Most job titles, while defined as to duties and responsibilities, are actually developed according to those already in the jobs. This is, in fact, how many human service workers have gotten footholds in local mental health systems, including state hospitals and mental health clinics. It is always easier to change an agency from within than to attack it frontally.

Because of the lack of specific job titles and job roles at many social service agencies, the budding human service worker should be warned about the inherent risks in establishing a human service beachhead. People and systems resist change. When confronted by a new way of doing something, they become suspicious and defensive. For the person who sees himself or herself as an agent of change, the result is usually the same: powerful forces within the system combine to drive the intruder out. Following are two case histories of persons who were motivated by a sense of responsibility to provide greater service—to change the system—and who, as a consequence were driven out.

Case History 1

The first story involves the struggle to develop and assert a meaningful job role for a group of mental health generalists at a state mental health center which was in the early stages of providing services to a larger group of patients than it had been serving before. The central figure in this story is a trainer whose job it was to hire, train, and implement a mental health, generalist group of trainees in the first of seven residential programs.

The trainer came to the institution with a general background in psychology, inservice treatment experience, and a commitment to help develop a new kind of mental health worker. At first, things went smoothly; a dozen new people were hired for the program. It was intended that they were to find jobs in the inpatient program along with personnel from other disciplines—psychiatrists, social workers, nurses, and rehabilitation counselors.

From the beginning, though, the trainer made several "political" mistakes: the trainees were isolated from the rest of the personnel, and communication was inhibited; the future role of the trainees was described as being that of generalists, people who would be able to do many different jobs; the trainees were encouraged to be critical of the roles and competence of the more traditional professionals; the trainer and his assistant were indiscreet—they gossiped about the top levels of the institution's administration without cautioning the trainees of the risks of spreading rumors; and the trainer became involved in a struggle with the director of training for the institution, both professionally and personally, over the issue of the director's competence and responsibility.

Then the director of training became the trainer's immediate boss, and struggle ensued between him, the trainer, the chief nurse, and the program-level administrators over the extent of the trainees' roles and responsibilities. The trainer lost in his bid to establish the trainees in a highly advantageous role in the program. As a result, they were left to muddle along for almost a year, until they were gradually accepted on the basis of personal ability.

301

The authors feel that many of the trainer's problems could probably have been avoided if he had not become embroiled in the struggle in such a personal way and if he had been more aware of, and able to respond to, the political pressures and factions of the agency. For example, he would probably have created less suspicion if he included other key administrators in the training process. This would have led the administrators to relate to the trainees as persons; Fred, Harry, Ruth, and Betty, rather than "that group of trouble makers." He and the group would probably have met with less resistance if they had not been as overtly critical of the more traditional disciplines, at least while they were most vulnerable. The trainer might have had an ally in the Director of Training rather than an overt enemy if he had tried to change her views and feelings rather than openly and publicly attacking her.

Case History 2

The key figure in the second story worked at a large state mental hospital which was and is entrenched in the medical model. He was hired as a psychologist, and on the basis of previous experience, was put in charge of a ward as its team leader. Previously he had worked in a pragmatic, mental health generalist style of operation at another agency program and had seen the results such a program could bring, in the way of service to patients and improved staff attitudes.

He began starting programs designed to improve the lives of long-term chronic patients. He expected his staff to become actively involved in all phases of the programs and invested much of his own time and energy, not only in working with the patients but in helping clean the ward, in attending night-shift meetings and encouraging the staff to find ways to help the long-term residents reenter the community.

All seemed to be going well. Initial staff resistance was overcome and replaced with enthusiasm about the program. The staff regarded their new team leader as being different from other administrators they had known. Their team leader was interested in the success of the program and was willing to go to bat for them if they had ideas that could improve service to the patients.

A few days before the team leader was to be certified (and thus gain civil service protection), he was called into the superintendent's

The human service worker today should be able to work with people from all walks of life and should be willing to do whatever is necessary to help the individual. (Courtesy Lexington School for the Deaf.)

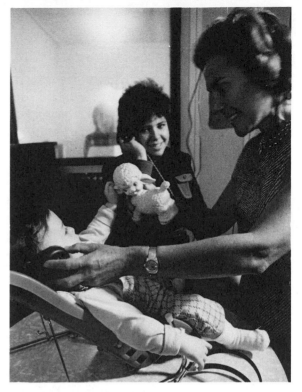

The preventive medicine of skilled work goes a long way. This boy in Casablanca is learning carpentry in an ORT school. (Courtesy Joint Distribution Committee.)

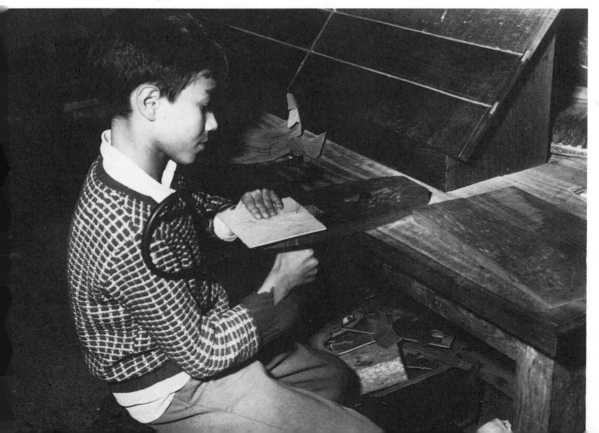

office and told that he was fired. The superintendent was so eager to see him leave that he was willing to pay the team leader's salary for the remainder of the fiscal year to any agency that would be willing to hire him.

In talking to him and others familiar with the situation, it was apparent that his behavior and willingness to try to improve the program were out of line with the expectancies of the agency's administrators. They had become concerned when they saw someone willing to work as a generalist in the human service model and struggle with solving problems and meeting real needs. His "mistake" had been to start doing his job before he had civil service protection.

University Training

The preparation for a human service job is not easy. In a paper by Walter Fisher, Robert Agranoff, Joseph Mehr, and Philip Truckenbrod, "The Service Agency and the University without Walls," we propose making university education more responsive to service agency needs by incorporating these themes:

The viewpoint of the service agencies must become part of the university curriculum.

Program primacy must be maintained, programs that can be applied to the needs, problems, and crises of the community rather than being harmonious with the training and needs of the care-giver.

The criterion for delivering services should be competence and not credentials.

Education and training should take place as close to the service area as possible.

It is not *where* you learn but *whether* you have learned the appropriate skills, information, and attitudes.

The task of the educator is not to lecture but to *identify* and *authenticate* those experiences that are educational. It is vital that this society stop routinely equating formal schooling with education.

A method should be found for giving academic credit for *all* learning experiences. As long as most employers continue to focus on college degrees as the criterion for employment, all "higher"-level learning experiences should be included in college transcripts.

Finally, most inservice training programs should become part of a university network and university credit should be given for them.

Summary

It seems clear that there are a multitude of jobs and functions which are involved in the task of helping the client. These can all be human service roles if they are approached with an attitude of working with the patient to solve problems and provide the kind of service which will lead the client to increased personal growth and expanded competencies. These job roles, if they do not formally exist, can be created by the person willing to implement the human service model.

The role of the human service worker is however a service delivery approach which is just beginning to make its impact felt across the country. There are each year many new college degree programs as well as inservice training efforts which are being developed to support and implement the human service worker.

As had been elaborated upon in previous chapters the needs of the client and our economy demand a new approach to providing services to all of the people, at all levels of society. The human service approach emphasizes the mobilization of all of the relevant resources available to a situation to insure that the client does not become linked into a career of dependency and poverty.

The growth of the human services is directly related to the energy, integrity, and ingenuity of the individual human service worker to bring the needed changes to the larger system.

Part V

A Glance into the Future

Chapter 20 A New Consciousness

In this book we have tried to identify a new enterprise called the *human services,* to relate it to social change, and to study its impact on the field of mental health. It should be clear by now that the human service approach goes well beyond the boundaries of mental health. It affects education, public health, penology, law enforcement, public aid—all of the social service systems.

In defining the human service approach in the field of mental health, we have compared it to the traditional mental health model (the Second Revolution's medical-Freudian model). We have compared the two models in terms of history, role, philosophy, organization, delivery systems, function, and training.

This last chapter will be used to present our perspective on mental health.

Belief I

The differences between the medical model and the human service model are more than the differences in technology, organization and delivery systems. In actuality, the differences can only be expressed in the level of awareness or consciousness of the caregiver. As stated earlier, to prepare a clinician for his career, he must be aided in gathering information, skills, and appropriate attitudes. However, one would support the concept that it is the attitudes, perception and level of consciousness that are the keys to the types and level of service.

In effect, it is being stated that if one summates the components of the medical model or the human service model, the sum of the parts are not equal to the whole of the model. That is, the model is more than the sum of the chapters of the book—it is a new gestalt (a new configuration).

Belief II

If one wanted to predict as to how an agency or a clinician would function, the main variables in contributing to the accuracy of such predictions would relate to the attitudes or perspective of the relevant individual or individuals (the level of consciousness).

In Western society, it has been the dominant motif to assume that if an individual is not functioning in an adaptive fashion, he is sick or diseased. The associative process to this theme is diagnosis, prognosis, finding the cause and cure. This is all to be done within the medical metaphor. If one pursues this motif, one ends up focusing on doctors, hospitals, treatment technologies, and vaccines. It is a highly structured, highly organized, and reasonably detailed configuration.

Belief III

The struggle between the human service model and the medical-Freudian model is not simply a struggle between professions attempting to determine the most effective service system. In effect, this struggle is a reflection of profound changes occurring in our society.

The society is in the midst of a transition from an industrial-wage society to a service supported society. Automation is a crucial factor in making this possible.

Less persons are required to provide the usual services in industry, farming, military service and all systems necessary to meet the basic needs of mankind.

Individuals who are employed are seeking job satisfactions beyond salary. Many more persons are no longer willing to work simply for a higher wage.

The disadvantaged persons in our society have greater expectancies and are more vocal in their demands for help. They are no longer willing to go into a corner and silently die.

It has become clear that the resources in the United States are not infinite. It is not possible to simply continue to expand budgets to meet the needs of public aid recipients, school children, mental health consumers, and all other social service clients. New initiatives and alternatives are required.

It is becoming increasingly clear that not all maladaptive persons are malfunctioning because of inner disorders. Many of the social systems and social institutions are malfunctioning and creating problems that the individual cannot resolve alone with his internal resources.

The emergence of the human service model (the Third Revolution) is an expression of changing patterns within the society. The United States has been traditionally dominated by the themes of the frontier, laissez faire economics, and rugged individualism. However, what happens to the many persons who, for a variety of reasons, cannot compete? As part of a survival of the fittest orientation, there is a tendency to perceive the failures as sick, lazy, or inferior. Some political leaders support a more planned society. In many ways, the planned society is an expression of the casualties produced by the competitive, survival of the fittest, highly individualistic free society. Just as such free societies produce "great men," it tends to increasingly produce disadvantaged persons: criminals, drug users, alcoholics, mental patients, socioeconomic failures, and scapegoated minorities. There is no question that as you plan your society to provide "first aid" and support for the "losers," you tend to interfere with the idealized "free market."

The authors feel the critical issues are expressed in the following questions:

How much of an investment does our society want to make in the disadvantaged persons? What are our national priorities?

Can it be assumed that the disadvantaged person has failed purely on the basis of his individualistic resources? Are the disadvantaged produced by the system?

Can the disadvantaged person be helped without modifying some of our basic social institutions: schools, families, churches, career patterns, prison, penal institutions, mental health facilities?

Can a highly competitive, highly individualistic, and goal oriented society aid its disadvantaged citizens without a major planned program?

Will competitive society tend to build an increasing residual population of disadvantaged persons? If so, what are the long term implications?

In effect, it is being suggested that the human service model has emerged as an option in order to respond to these national problems.

Belief IV

In Belief III, there was an attempt to establish the cultural context for the human service model. The human service theme appears to the authors to be a national issue, in effect, a cabinet post issue. It can be assumed that all cultural units have something akin to a "gross deviance." That is, in regard to any country we can speak of a "Gross National Deviance (G.N.D.)." The configuration of this G.N.D. is predicated on national priorities: employment rates, resource distribution, laws, political organization, and international affairs.

If one truly wanted to alter a deviance pattern, it would require the altering of the national priorities. This approach can better be understood if the addiction problem (drugs and alcohol) is briefly examined. As long as the authors can remember, there have been attempts to resolve the problem: Alcoholics Anonymous, Synanon, antibuse, psychoanalysis, education, and chemical substitutions (heroin for the opiates and methadone for heroin).

It seems very clear as one examines the national scene that there has been no reduction in these problems. In fact, the problem has increased over the last few years. The task of temporarily removing the individual from the addictive substance is not the difficult problem. Clinicians know that can be done quite easily. It is providing a viable and meaningful substitution for the addictive substance. The following pattern can be seen rather frequently. An individual is released from a mental health residential unit as "cured" from his alcoholism. He returns to a society in which he has typically adjusted in a maladaptive way. The options are the same aversive patterns: same old friends, same old unskilled job, same old pains, and same old sex life. It is possible that alcohol may be the only reasonable solution under these circumstances. If service givers are unable to link persons to new life styles that are exciting and meaningful, then service agencies might just as well forget about resolving the addiction problems. This brings us to the following questions:

How much money is society willing to expend on resolving the addiction problem?

What national priorities is our society willing to alter to aid the addiction problem?

How serious a national problem is addiction?

Why does society continue to perpetuate the problem?

Addiction, like most other human problems that we have labeled—for example, schizophrenia, manic depressive and sociopathic—are issues that emerge from the main fabric of our society. They are products of the alienation and unlinking that most societies produce. It is naive to assume that mental health workers functioning in private practice, clinics and hospitals are going to relink and reintegrate the enormous multitude of malfunctioning people in our society.

societal institutions on producing deviance. To resolve these questions it will require decisions at the federal level in order to decrease our G.N.D.

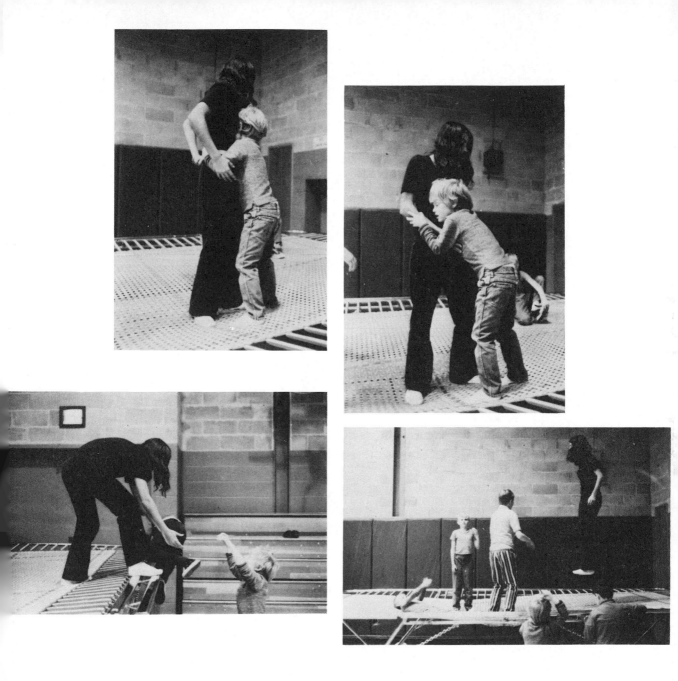

Many patients have great expectations and are vocal in their
demands for help. (Photos by Costa Manos, courtesy Magnum.)

Belief V

It appears to suit the national conscience to assume that most deviant behavior is a function of a disease process. People are labeled schizophrenic, manic depressive, and sociopathic, and then the labelers attempt to establish the causes as faulty genes, poor blood chemistry, or metabolic disorders. The alleged disease processes are then left in the hands of the professionals. In effect, this extrudes the deviant persons from our society. One can malfunction as a result of genes, blood chemistry problems, and disorders in metabolism, but most maladaptations are a function of the impact of the social systems and social institutions on the individual. The malfunctioning citizen is a cultural casualty—a consequence of a societal style.

Belief VI

As one begins the process of expanding one's consciousness in regard to the issues of mental health, the precept of a patient obsessively searching for his problems and solutions on an analyst's couch at $50 per session appears extremely trivial. It is not so much that one should oppose this process as attempt to develop a sense of proportion and appropriate national priorities. The patient on the couch, in terms of our Gross National Deviances, represents one minor option among many.

Belief VII

It is preferable to avoid the concept that people are sick or are not sick. The concept of normality appears to be a cultural expression of utopia—a hoped for idealistic state. The orientation of this book is pragmatic and practical. The authors are suggesting that there are a wide variety of styles of life which have different degrees of congruence with the main cultural patterns. When one refers to styles of life, it is a referral to a pattern of traits, values, interests, philosophies and beliefs. For a more comprehensive review of this concept of styles of life, we would suggest the following references: Walter Fisher (1965), Melanie Klein (1949) and Eric Erikson (1963).

It is being hypothesized that some styles of life are more adaptive to particular cultural styles. Therefore certain individuals might do better in nineteenth century America and others might be more successful in the latter part of the twentieth century. That is, contingent upon the cultural or national priorities, different life styles might be more or less effective in a particular society at a particular time in history.

The question before the mental health caregiver is not whether an individual is ill but what services might be needed. It is a decision making process. Examples of possible services:

No services.

The client can remain at home and only needs counseling.

Day hospital or night hospital services.

Linking services (job, career series, cash economy, social organization, integrity group).

Residential care.

In effect, the service giver develops an understanding of the individual's life style and attempts to link the person with those services that will allow the individual to function adequately or cope within his environment. This appears preferable to labeling or name-calling.

Belief VIII

It is a major task of the caregiver to begin to understand the impact of social institutions and social systems on the various life styles extant in our culture. The authors of this book have in previous writings (1973a), (1973b) and (1973c) referred to the concept, Treatment Through Institutional Change.

This theme is that much of human behavior—adaptive and maladaptive—is determined by various social institutions and systems acting upon individuals at any one time. For most people, their schools, careers, church, and family have a continuous impact on their immediate behavior. If service givers are indeed to help people—provide antidotes for their maladaptation—it is important to understand the various influences of social institutions on different life styles. In order to serve people. human service workers must be prepared to develop new social institutions or modify old ones.

EXAMPLES:

Problems	*Solutions*
Addicts do not respond to professional mental health workers.	The use of former addicts as therapists; e.g., Alcoholics Anonymous and Synanon.
Many persons seeking education do not find it in the traditional classrooms.	There is the recent development of the "university without walls."
Persons are locked into jobs and are unable to move up the socio-economic ladder.	The development of the career series.
The failure of the family and church in relinking persons back into the mainstream of society.	The development of integrity or peer groups.

It seems that mental health workers should develop expertise in identifying and influencing those social institutions that aid members of the society in becoming more adaptive.

Belief IX

The major task of caregivers is identifying and authenticating those experiences by which people grow or mature. The traditional therapy experiences:: free association, insight, interpretation, dream analysis, transference and searching through someone's past, might have provided growth experiences for the highly motivated, mainstream, middle-class client but they are ineffective with most disadvantaged persons.

The primary target population for the mental health worker in today's society is the maladaptive person who rejects traditional help systems and yet requires help if he is to stay out of institutions. These are the persons who have been limited to state hospitals and prison as "growth experiences."

Every culture and subculture has an elaborate behavioral modification pattern that influences and determines the behavior of those in the culture. If you perform in the appropriate fashion, you are rewarded, and, of course, if you perform in an inappropriate fashion, you are punished. The power structure in every society designs the behavior modification matrix that rewards and punishes the members of the society. It is not a consciously formalized or written code of behavior but an implicit, emotional subthreshold and ever present system. Ultimately, this behavior modification model tends to influence everyone to behave like the power structure.

The school model game is an excellent example of this behavior-modification scheme. Some children from the day they enter school accept the school game: good grades, swallow information, be a good child, listen to the teacher, go as far in school as possible, school equals competence, school is the elevator to the "top" and everyone should want to go there. If you can and want to pursue this game, the society will reward you and generally, despite the negative effects of this processing system, the individual will receive life long rewards: good income, good housing, good career and security.

If the schooling process does not turn you on, what happens? There will be a history of poor grades, truancy, the development of a negative self-image and rather frequently a career of failure. It is known that many minority groups and various persons emerging from disadvantaged families never get inspired by our public school systems. This is definitely not their game plan.

In the school model there is an example of a social institution that provides growth experience for certain members of our society and yet for others, it results in destructive and regressive experiences. In effect, for many generations, most persons have passively and implicitly accepted the notion that if one fails in public school, he really should not be successful and that he should remain at the bottom of a career level. Alienation, maladaptation and deviance are built into the model.

It becomes the task of human service workers to understand the impact of social institutions, positive and negative, to identify and authenticate these impacts and attempt to provide options. Those persons who cannot use traditional schools can be provided with other options by which they can grow. If we only provide reform schools, prisons and mental hospitals, then society can be prepared to receive an alienated, maladaptive and violent product. It is only in recent years that writers, such as Ivan Illich (1970), have begun to attempt to provide options to the traditional school system.

Belief X

It is important that human service systems remain flexible, open and constantly available to change. Helping people, at this point in history, is typically not a scientific endeavor. It is more related to values, politics, problem solving, pragmatism and interpersonal skills. The new human service worker should be constantly seeking more efficient and effective models.

There was a time when mental health workers assumed insight could be equated with "cure." There is no evidence available to support this contention. In fact, many experienced clinicians will tell you that insight might do as much harm as good. There are many clinical reports that insight can frequently lead to regression or suicide.

Recently, one of the authors of this book was interviewing a patient who was diagnosed as having grand mal seizures and being extremely paranoid. It reminded him of a myth that epileptics never become psychotic. This was one of the rationales for the shock therapies.

In recent years, the number of persons in state hospitals have been massively reduced. As one looks through these case folders of released patients, it is amazing to see how many of them were considered to have a hopeless prognosis. Many of the traditional caregivers did not realize that the prognostic statements on the patients were really statements on the limitation of their treatment models.

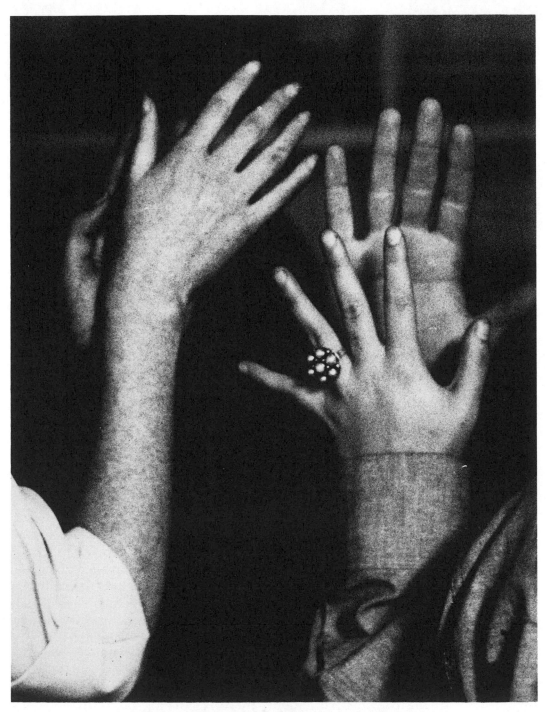

The greatest contribution of the third revolution in mental health is the concept of *helping* the individual as a unique person. (Photo by Costa Manos, courtesy Magnum.)

There are endless mental health myths that were equated with truths.

Myths:

It is possible to identify and define a pattern that we can label mental illness.

Insulin shock therapy will cure mental illness.

The caregiver has to understand the cause of the mental illness to help a person.

Only physicians can treat mentally ill persons.

If a person thinks he is mentally ill, he really isn't ill.

Suicide is a defense against homicide.

If you find the cause of an illness, you will "cure" the person.

There are experts who can predict homicide and suicide.

There is a relationship between diagnosis and treatment utilized.

There are endless myths, unsubstantiated beliefs, in the mental health field. It is not that one should completely abandon all of these beliefs, ideas, concepts and notions. The problem is to evaluate and determine their effectiveness and pursue more effective alternatives.

Summary

It is assumed the boundaries of the human service field are extensive, the content massive, and the system constantly expanding. The major task of this book is to sensitize the reader to the task. One cannot aid a client by means of a network of theories. A client needing help is a here and now phenomenon. The service giver has to mature to the point that he is able to identify the problem and the service needed and expedite or deliver the service. In a sense, each time a worker delivers service it is a unique event, so in this context, the service giver can only rely upon what he has to deliver as a person. You cannot bring Freud or any other service giver into the service situation with you. You are there, and in some way must know what you are capable of bringing to the client.

320

In the previous statement, there is nothing being taken away from the service giver; instead it is an attempt to identify the services and skills that any individual has to provide. It is not clear what experiences result in the mental health worker's development of competencies. The role of the educational system in creating competence is unclear. The individual's service capability may be primarily a matter of the personal equation factor (appearance, intelligence and emotional patterns). The authors feel the personal equation factors are crucial in the delivery of service based on their experiences and observations.

Perhaps some persons will find these final statements anxiety producing or depressing, but there are other ways of experiencing these concepts. Seeking to help people without strict formal guidelines is an exciting quest. It becomes the task of the caregiver to become aware of available resources and to utilize them in a creative fashion. The potential for resourcefulness, initiative, and creativity supercedes most fields of endeavor. The creativity lies in identifying growth experiences and providing effective configurations of service. The ultimate creativity is in assessing your personal potential to provide services.

Appendix: Program Development Manual

CONTENTS

Introduction to Elgin State Hospital
Program Development Project

In an effort to support the planning and development of new treatment programs, staff development has looked about for alternatives to the traditional approaches to training. The traditional approach, utilizing classroom and blackboard techniques, must be reexamined in the face of its inability to involve the participants and bring about change in the larger institution. It is all too apparent that there are only a very few charismatic individuals who can effectively use the classroom to deliver the kind and quality of training that a large institution urgently needs. It is obvious that the classroom must be largely abandoned in spite of a given teacher's ability or student's commitment, in favor of a new vehicle for the delivery of training. Ideally the training vehicle should have the following qualities:

1. It must increase the participation of all persons involved in the process.
2. It must abandon caste concepts such as *student, trainee, teacher,* and *lecturer,* and replace them with the expectation that everyone involved in the learning experience has a contribution to make.
3. It must have as a site, a place where actual ongoing problems and processes can be encountered and dealt with.
4. The training experience should simultaneously involve all of the members of a treatment team. This strategy helps to counter problems arising when one or two employees are trained and then return to the ward where their enthusiasm is diluted by the inertia of the ongoing program.

In an attempt to include some of the above design features in a training experience which involves the entire treatment team, the following program development training is suggested:

324

1. Treatment teams will be identified which are committed

to working toward a service delivery system designed to meet identified goals and objectives.

2. Each participating team will recruit a coach from another area of the hospital, who will keep the team in touch with the problem and provide suggestions, alternatives, and on-the-job experience. The coaches will be senior staff persons who have had experience in developing and implementing programs.

3. Consultants with special skills in program development or organizational systems will be made available to the teams, and they will be matched with the team's goals and objectives.

4. Staff development, in coordination with program area training coordinators, will provide the consultants, resources, and general management for the entire project and insure that persons are given training credit.

5. Meetings will include:
  (a) intrateam meetings with the coach
  (b) team meetings with consultants
  (c) meetings with the coaches
  (d) interteam meetings
  (e) meeting of coaches, consultants, and program directors

6. Consultation will be provided to develop methods of evaluating the changes in the service delivery system as a result of the new program, in the context of the team's stated goals and objectives.

7. Each team will prepare a paper describing the process and changes.

8. Teams and coaches will be used in future program development training to help other teams.

Contained in this manual are (1) a three-phase flowchart of operations which the team will follow, (2) a workbook with operation objectives and team process documentation, (3) a coach subroutine, (4) a task group subroutine, and (5) a glossary of project terms.

The training package can initially have six to nine hours of college credit tied to it. Plans are underway to develop a complete undergraduate program with the Program Development Training Project being used for one of the four years as the major area of concentration.

The Program Development Training Project is a system designed to deliver training to the treatment programs themselves. Its advantages include an ability to involve the team members in training which is directly connected with their regular job activities, increasing treatment program effectiveness, and upgrading staff skills around the program treatment modalities. This type of a training delivery system allows the treatment program to participate and implement training programs to meet their own needs. This project will make it possible to support and encourage the development of well-designed programs through the use of course work, program consultants, and workshops. As a result, treatment programs will have an increased capacity to meet the needs of their primary group of patients. It is anticipated that as a result of this program there will be many benefits relating to the overall institution's ability to respond to the human service needs of the communities it serves.

Program Development Project: Workbook

Description

The purpose of this workbook is to give each team a set of guidelines with which to pursue its goal of creating a new program.

Each numbered item below is related to a numbered block on the flowcharts which are included. Within the numbered item are four subdivisions which will be briefly described here:

A. *Objectives of each operation.* An outline of the processes the team needs to deal with.

B. *Team specific objectives.* An agenda developed by the team for the meeting. It may be arrived at before the meeting or in the early stages of the meeting. It amounts to an operationalizing of the guidelines established in A above.

C. *Behavioral description of team activities.* Semi-detailed notes on each meeting. While they need not be verbatim notes, they should reflect the meeting's atmosphere, chronology, issues, and problems.

D. *Evaluation Activity.* A retrospective discussion of the conclusions the team has reached in the course of each operation and the considerations which led them to these decisions. The logic which defined the next step in program development should be identified and analyzed. This item entails a conscientious look at the team's decision-making process during this step and a justification of the conclusions.

The completion of this manual should be a team endeavor, one in which the entire team is directly involved. At the end of each meeting, the workbook page corresponding to the operation in which the team is involved should be completed. One copy of this document will be for Staff Development's records, one for the coach and consultant, one for the team's records, and one for the program director.

It might be wise to appoint a secretary for all meetings as one of the first operations of the team process.

Phase 1: Identification of Problems, Goals, and Objectives

Objective of the Operation:

1. (a) The entire team reaches a consensus on the need for a new program. Relevant options for new program development are discussed. The Program Development Training Project is presented and discussed. The team decides that the Program Development Training Project is the best option available for the development of a new program. The team representatives contact the staff development to enlist.

(b) *team specific objectives*

(c) *behavioral description of team activities*

(d) *evaluation activity*

327

Objective of the Operation:

2. (a) The team recruits a coach who is a member of the senior staff from another area of the hospital. The coach is selected on the basis of his experience in program development problems and the positive regard the team has for him. He is not selected on the basis of his specialized knowledge in a specific treatment technique. The team will develop a set of practical goals and objectives for the program to be developed. In a sense, they will define why the ward program exists. By this time, a secretary should have been selected.

(b) *team specific objectives*

(c) *behavioral description of team activities*

(d) *evaluation activity*

Objective of the Operation:

3. (a) The team decides whether they are prepared to initiate specific planning for the design of the new program. All technological and organizational issues must be resolved by now.

(b) *team specific objectives*

(c) *behavioral description of team activities*

(d) *evaluation activity*

Objective of the Operation:

4. (a) The team must examine its status and decide what its primary problem is: technology or organization. It is likely that the team will have to examine both areas in depth before it will be ready to go on to actual planning for a new program.

(b) *team specific objectives*

(c) *behavioral description of team activities*

(d) *evaluation activity*

Objective of the Operation

5. (a) The team, or its designates, a task group, undertakes an inventory of all mental health technology related to their case-specific problems and to their goals and objectives. The technological skills of the team are surveyed and inventoried. By the end of this operation, the team should know how much resource acquisition in the area of technology they will have to perform.

(b) *team specific objectives*

(c) *behavioral description of team activities*

(d) *evaluation activity*

Ojective of the Operation:

6. (a) The team or its designates, a task group, examine their organizational structure to determine whether or not they can adapt to a new program which will place other demands on them and on the individual members of the team. Roles will have to be examined and resistance to change dealt with. New and broader role definitions will be developed in some cases.

(b) *team specific objectives*

(c) *behavioral description of team activities*

(d) *evaluation activity*

Objective of the Operation:

7. (a) The team decides whether its organizational and technological problems are resolved. Is the team unable to translate its organization into treatment? Are interpersonal issues impossible to deal with?

(b) *team specific objectives*

(c) *behavioral description of team activities*

(d) *evaluation activity*

Objective of the Operation:

8. (a) Have final attempts to resolve organizational and technological problems been reasonably successful? Are the new organizational arrangements acceptable to a majority of the team? Have suitable new roles been established and accepted? Is the team's organizational structure now sound enough to deal with the demands of a new treatment program? Have treatment options been inventoried?

   (b) *team specific objectives*

   (c) *behavioral description of team activities*

   (d) *evaluation activity*

Objective of the Operation:

9. (a) Team prepares for entry into Phase II, Designing a New Game Plan. The team will review Phase I to determine whether or not it is satisfied with its work and will initiate the alternate game plan development.

   (b) *team specific objectives*

   (c) *behavioral description of team activities*

   (d) *evaluation activity*

Phase II: Designing A New Game Plan

Objective of the Operation:

10. (a) The team examines and discusses the game plans presented to it. What are their implications? Which best suits the particular ward's circumstances?

(b) *team specific objectives*

(c) *behavioral description of team activities*

(d) *evaluation activity*

Objective of the Operation:

11. (a) Has the task group been able to deliver suitable alternate game plans? If it has not, the task group should be given direct team feedback on what is required. The team should discuss the problem in order to ascertain exactly why none of the alternate game plans was acceptable. Has the team encountered unforeseeable technological or organizational problems?

(b) *team specific objectives*

(c) *behavioral description of team activities*

(d) *evaluation activity*

Objective of the Operation:

12. (a) The team has not found an acceptable alternate game plan; return to operation 4 of Phase I for further preprogram development problem-solving.

(b) *team specific objectives*

(c) *behavioral description of team activities*

(d) *evaluation activity*

Objective of the Operation:

13. (a) The team chooses a basic game plan structure. Preliminary work on implementation is begun with discussions of how to turn the basic structure into the most effective treatment program. Staff development helps team in securing consultant. The coach, consultant and staff development meet with the program director to discuss progress and to plan for future development.

(b) *team specific objectives*

(c) *behavioral description of team activities*

(d) *evaluation activity*

333

Objective of the Operation:

14. (a) Detailed game plan implementation options are brought to the team by task groups. These options might include rough schedules, ward organizations, role definitions, materials acquisition lists, and possible training needs. The team then decides on an implementation from the options offered.

(b) *team specific objectives*

(c) *behavioral description of team activities*

(d) *evaluation activity*

Objective of the Operation:

15. (a) If the task groups are unable to present suitable implementations for the basic game plan, the team will undergo a thorough review of the assumptions and processes which have caused the failure. Can an implementation be devised? Is the basic game plan faulty?

(b) *team specific objectives*

(c) *behavioral description of team activities*

(d) *evaluation activity*

Phase III: Training and Implementation

Objective of the Operation:

16. (a) At this time, the team begins to create task groups to deal with specific aspects of the game plan implementation. All or most of the conceptual issues should have been dealt with by now.

(b) *team specific objectives*

(c) *behavioral description of team activities*

(d) *evaluation activity*

Objective of the Operation:

17. (a) Training needs should be identified specifically. Task groups can serve the team in the accumulation and organization of this data in consultation with the area training coordinator and staff development coaches and consultants.

(b) *team specific objectives*

(c) *behavioral description of team activities*

(d) *evaluation activity*

Objective of the Operation:

18. (a) The team and/or task groups make a final effort to identify and analyze training needs. **A** basic decision must be made by the team as to whether or not, given the game plan and implementation, the training needs can be analyzed, identified, or met.

(b) *team specific objectives*

(c) *behavioral description of team activities*

(d) *evaluation activity*

Objective of the Operation:

19. (a) The team has been unable to identify or analyze training needs. Return to operation 14 in Phase II.

(b) *team specific objectives*

(c) *behavioral description of team activities*

(d) *evaluation activity*

Objective of the Operation:

20. (a) A suitable training program must be designed and implemented on the ward. It must be all-inclusive, that is, aim toward

training all team members. It must be specific in the goals it hopes to attain. An acting training coordinator, or training task group, might be chosen to arrange and supervise the special ward training, or the regular area training coordinator might be contacted to help. The goal of this is to bring all team members up to about the same level of program competency.

(b) *team specific objectives*

(c) *behavioral description of team activities*

(d) *evaluation activity*

Objective of the Operation:

21. (a) Operation 21 specifies a number of functions the team must accomplish before moving beyond this point. Each is essential to the successful initiation of the program. Also, the program must be started at this time. The team will meet to examine the fledgling program. Problems will be openly examined and solved. Any minor alterations or improvements will be planned and implemented. Additional or corrective training will be arranged and conducted. Current program operation will be discussed in light of the goals and objectives the team outlined in operation 2.

(b) *team specific objectives*

(c) *behavioral description of team activities*

(d) *evaluation activity*

337

Objective of the Operation:

22. (a) The team, coach, consultant, and staff development meet with the program director to discuss the program. Any objections to the program are raised and discussed.

(b) *team specific objectives*

(c) *behavioral description of team activities*

(d) *evaluation activity*

Objective of the Operation:

23. (a) A task group is assigned to write a final documentation of the project. This will be a detailed document, relying heavily on the notes taken during meetings, which will present all operations of the team. Planning, problem-solving, attitudes, development, training, implementation, and operation of the new program are discussed.

(b) *team specific objectives*

(c) *behavioral description of team activities*

(d) *evaluation activity*

Objective of the Operation:

24. (a) Ongoing team meetings are instituted to review the operation of the program. These meetings provide a continuous upkeep and adjustment of the program.

    (b) *team specific objectives*

    (c) *behavioral description of team activities*

    (d) *evaluation activity*

Objective of the Operation:

25. (a) End of program development phase.

    (b) *team specific objectives*

    (c) *behavioral description of team activities*

    (d) *evaluation activity*

Coach Subroutine

The coach is a voluntary member of the team who performs a variety of different functions. He serves the team in a consulting role, helping them through difficult periods with advice, counseling, and suggestions. He is to see that the team keeps its task in mind. He gives advice whenever it seems suitable but avoids directing the team. He bears in mind that a significant benefit of the project is that the team itself will work together to solve its problems.

The coach attends as many team and task group meetings as possible, preferably all. He also maintains contact with staff development, sending them a short written summary of each team or task force meeting. This summary is primarily his evaluation of how well the team performed its task. (These summaries will be used in the documentation of the team's Program Development Training Project.)

The coach assumes responsibility for seeing that the intent of the Program Development Training Project is carried out.

The team and the coach should work out a contract in the initial stages of the project, specifying the details of the relationship the coach will have with the team. Such details as time commitment, scheduling of meetings, rides, and personal agendas, will be established at this time.

Task Group Subroutine

The task group is a designated team subgroup, composed of no less than three team members, representing insofar as is possible each job classification and each shift. Its function is to accumulate and organize information according to the instructions of the team.

A task group may be appointed by the team whenever the team decides that a decision will require too much initial processing of information for the team as a whole to effectively deal with. The task group will then facilitate the acquisition and organization of pertinent information for the use of the team.

The task group may be called on by the team to develop a set of options, but it may not select an option for the team; it has no executive function.

Any given task group may be assigned no more than one limited task. In no circumstances may a single task group perform its duties in consecutive operations. A task group is an ad hoc body, which is created for a specific function. It ceases to exist as soon as that function is completed or if the team wishes to disband it before completion of its task for any reason.

Task group membership should be rotated so that in the course of the project, as many people as possible will have the opportunity to serve in a task group. Where two separate tasks are related, an overlap between the membership of the previous task group and the new task group is not only permitted but advisable.

Program Development Glossary

Coach A senior staff person from an area of the hospital other than that in which the team works, who has expertise in the development of new programs and is not to be selected solely on the basis of any specialized knowledge of treatment modalities.

Consultant A person with a specialized knowledge in organizational systems or program development who will help the team set up their program.

Evaluation The process of examining the team's activities and judging to what extent they are in line with the team's goals and objectives. Evaluation takes place at three levels: a) at the end of each operation, b) at the conclusion of the program development, and c) as an ongoing team function after the end of the project.

Game Plan The skeletal structure around which a new program is built. A game plan may be the basic treatment modality to be used in the new program, or it may be a well-defined orientation to the delivery of services (e.g., to keep the patients occupied and involved 12 hours a day).

Goals and Objectives The team's own definition of what its task is. This definition should *not* attempt to narrowly delineate a treatment program. It *should* outline an orientation to care delivery which will guide the team's activities in the future.

341

Operation The basic unit which defines a set of related tasks that must be achieved before any future tasks can be undertaken.

Organization The complex of relationship, both official and unofficial, which determine the manner in which any group sets about achieving its goals and objectives.

Phase A set of directly related operations, in which each phase is an integral component of the project and which must be completed before beginning the next phase.

Program A set of activities pursued by an organization of persons, based on a common set of goals, objectives, and tasks.

Program Development Training Project A system designed to facilitate program reorganization and introduce training directly onto the treatment ward.

Resource A unit of information or material that will support program development, also individuals or organizations which will provide these items.

Role A set of behaviors, or the perception of that set, which define an individual's relationship to other persons, groups, and organizations.

Task Group A team subgroup created to perform a specified task when the team decides it is not feasible to adequately perform in plenary session.

Team An organization of persons whose existence owes itself to goals and objectives related to mental health service delivery.

Glossary

acting out   Exhibiting problems in overt behavior, rather than controlling them via suppression or other defenses.

addiction   Physical dependence on drugs or alcohol.

adjustment   The relationship between an individual and his coping with his environment.

affect   Any experience of emotion or feeling.

aftercare   The follow-up of clients or patients discharged from agencies in an attempt to prevent their readmission.

aggression   The tendency to attack rather than withdraw or compromise in the face of stress; may or may not involve hostility.

anxiety   Vague tension or fear.

assumption   A statement accepted or supposed true without proof, demonstration, or evidence.

attitude   The tendency to respond with positive or negative emotion to certain persons, objects, or situations.

bedlam   The popular contraction of the name of the early London asylum of St. Mary of *Bethlehem;* refers to chaotic conditions.

343

behavior   Any observable action or set of responses of a person or animal.

behavior, deviant   Behavior that is significantly different from the social norm.

behavior disorder   A general term referring to psychoneurotic reactions, psychotic reactions, character and personality disorders, and chronic brain syndromes; means about the same as mental illness, though the logic is clearer.

behaviorism   The point of view that psychology is limited to the study of observable behavior.

behavior therapy   A form of psychotherapy which focuses on changing the problem behavior by using techniques of respondent, operant, and observational learning; similar in meaning to behavior modification.

belief   Acceptance of the validity of a statement; the thought portion of an attitude.

brain syndrome, chronic   Behavior disorders caused by long-lasting disturbances in brain function.

career ladder or series   A policy which allows the employees of an agency to be promoted to increasing levels of responsibility based on competence.

catchment area   Delivery of mental health services by geographic area.

catharsis   Discharge of emotional tension associated with repressed traumatic material by "talking it out"; may be achieved during interview therapy or by hypnosis or drugs such as sodium amytal.

cerebellum   The structure in the hindbrain which controls the coordination of movements and balance.

chemotherapy   Treatment of a psychoneurotic or a psychotic reaction with a chemical substance.

client-centered therapy   A nondirective therapy developed by Carl Rogers that typically is neither as intensive nor as prolonged as psychoanalysis.

conditioning, classical   Learning that takes place when a conditioned stimulus is paired with an unconditioned stimulus.

consumerism   A new spirit of the times which leads people to demand and lobby for good products, effective services, and honesty.

control   The group in an experiment which is similar in all respects to the experimental group, with the exception of the treatment condition.

coping behavior   Attempting to adjust to problems by seeking solutions.

crisis   An extremely emotional, temporary state during which a person loses his normal capacity to interact with his environment.

criterion   In the evaluation of tests, the job or level of performance that test is supposed to predict.

culture   Customs, habits, traditions, and objects that characterize a people or a social group; includes the attitudes and beliefs the group has about important aspects of its life.

culture pattern   Widely shared beliefs and ways of behaving in a society.

daytop   A small group residential treatment approach to drug dependency.

delivery system   A general strategy for bringing services to a group of patients, for example, a comprehensive community mental health clinic.

deviance, cultural   Abnormal patterns of social organization, attitudes, or behavior; undesirable social conditions which tend to produce individual pathology.

diagnosis   Determination of the nature and extent of a disorder.

disenfranchisement   The cutting off of a person in crisis from the important aspects of his environment, social and physical, which tend to support his normal ability to cope.

disorientation   Confusion with respect to time, place, or person.

drive   The motive power behind behavior.

Durham Rule   The legal interpretation of insanity that held that the defendant is not held criminally responsible for his behavior if he has a mental illness or defect.

economy   Financial resources available to an agency.

economy, principle of   The concept that the individual meets stress in the simplest way possible: in terms of his evaluation of the stress situation and of his own capacities.

economy, token   Behavior modification technique used with groups; similar to the capitalistic form of economics, with tokens serving the function of money.

electroconvulsive shock therapy (ECT)   A form of therapy used primarily with depressed patients. It involves administering electrical shocks to the forebrain sufficient to produce convulsion.

elitist   A professional with a great deal of credentials and experience.

etiology   Causation; the systematic study of the causes of disorders.

evaluation, environmental   The way in which the individual views the world, its dangers, and so forth.

exorcism   The driving out of evil spirits through prayer or physical punishment of the "possessed" individual.

expedite   To facilitate, or help, a process.

extended care A service delivery system designed to deal with the chronic patient.

feedback A situation in which some aspect of the output regulates the state of the system; a form of reinforcement from the learning viewpoint.

flowchart A "progress map" which defines the operations the team can and will take in the completion of its task.

foster home Usually a home consisting of a family which takes in short-term placements of nonfamily members, most often children.

free association Psychoanalytic technique of having a patient say whatever comes to his mind, regardless of how irrelevant or objectionable it may seem on the surface.

Freudian Based on the theories of Sigmund Freud.

frustration Thwarting of a need or desire.

functional In reference to behavior disorders, having no demonstrable organic cause or etiology; also known as psychogenic.

game plan The skeletal structure around which a new program is built; may be the basic treatment to be used in a new program or a well-defined orientation to the delivery of services (e.g., to keep patients occupied and involved 12 hours a day).

garbage dump An institution where a person is placed which offers few experiences to help him function independently.

generalist One who performs some work of all types, in contrast to a specialist who performs more restricted work.

gerontology The study of old age.

gestalt therapy A technique designed to help a person confront himself and the discrepancies in his perceptions and relations with himself and other people.

goals and objectives An agency's definition of its task.

group therapy Discussion of personal problems by a group of patients under the guidance of a therapist; may take a variety of forms, depending on the theoretical orientation of the therapist.

halfway house A treatment site in the community.

Hawthorne effect The introduction of anything into group functioning that subsequently increases group effectiveness and performance.

hierarchy A group of entities arranged according to a graded system such as rank, authority, or importance.

homeostasis A state of equilibrium produced by a balance of functions.

human service model Delivery of services characterized by a pragmatic style of problem-solving with an emphasis on the solving of the current and most urgent problems.

human services   The broad area of providing helping services of all sorts to human beings. It subsumes the areas of mental health, corrections, welfare education, etc., and includes both formal and informal organizations and networks.

hydrotherapy   Use of hot or cold baths, ice packs, etc., in the treatment of mental patients.

hyperactivity   Disturbed behavior, usually of children, which results from some type of minimal brain damage or immaturity.

hypochondriac   One whose neurosis is characterized by an excessive concern over his health in the absense of concrete symptoms.

hypochondriasis   Neurotic reaction characterized by an excessive concern about one's health in the absence of related physical illness.

hypothesis   An assertion, subject to verification as a conjecture, which accounts for a set of facts within an ideational framework and which can be used as a basis for further investigation.

hysteria   An older term which includes conversion and dissociative neurotic reactions; involves the simulation of symptoms of organic illness in the absence of any related organic pathology.

insane   A legal term for a mental disorder accompanied by lack of responsibility for one's acts.

insight   In psychotherapy, the understanding of one's own motives and their origins.

instinct   An inherited response.

institution   Ideally a complex system for managing and expediting human behavior.

integrity group   A small group approach for individuals who are attempting to face their problems and accept responsibility for them.

intraorganismic   Pertaining to the internal functioning and processes of an organism.

involutional psychosis   Agitated depression or paranoid reactions in women at menopause, considerably influenced by psychological factors.

lesbian   A woman who prefers homosexual to bisexual encounters.

leucotomy   A brain operation involving the severing of association pathways in the frontal lobes of the brain, in which the instruments are inserted transorbitally rather than by drilling holes in the top or sides of the skull.

lobectomy   A psychosurgery technique.

lobotomy   A surgical procedure involving the separation of neurofibers between the frontal and other regions of the brain. In the past it was believed that the operation led to a decrease in abnormal behavior. The procedure is less commonly used today because it is of doubtful benefit.

lunacy   A legal term roughly synonymous with insanity.

madness   An old term referring to severe mental illness.

maladaptive   The process of not effectively adapting.

malinger   To consciously fake illness or disability symptoms.

McNaghten Rule   A legal interpretation of insanity which basically asks whether a person is able to distinguish between right and wrong.

medical model   The model of treating mental illness characterized by the diagnose, treat, and cure approach modeled after the treatment of physical disorders such as polio.

mental disease   Mental disorder associated with an organic disease of the nervous system, e.g., syphilis of the nervous system.

mental health system   An organization of services designed to provide care for persons exhibiting deviant behavior usually called mental illness.

mental health technologies   Methods and techniques used to improve the behavioral condition of disturbed people; includes individual and group counseling or therapy, chemotherapy, education, and remotivation.

mental health worker   A term which may pertain to any of the traditional mental health professionals, although it is more commonly used in reference to individuals with less formal education, including those who have Associate in Arts degrees in mental health technology and related areas.

mesmerism   Relating to the theories of "animal magnetism" (hypnosis) formulated by Anton Mesmer.

metrazol therapy   The administration of metrazol to produce epileptiform convulsions; formerly used in the treatment of certain psychotic reactions.

microcosm   A system similar to a much larger system.

milieu therapy   An approach which seeks to make a person both responsive to and interactive with his environment.

model   A conceptual framework of persons, roles, values, technologies, and philosophies for delivering mental health services.

mores   Customs that enforce social values having ethical or moral significance; violation brings strong social disapproval.

motivation, unconscious   Motivation that can be inferred from the person's behavior but which cannot be verbalized by the person himself.

neo-Freudian   Based on the theories of later, nontraditional students of Sigmund Freud.

nervous breakdown A popular term denoting neurotic or psychotic levels of personality decompensation.

neurosis A mild functional personality disorder.

obsession Seemingly irrational idea that constantly intrudes into a person's thoughts.

obsessive-compulsive reaction Psychoneurotic reaction characterized by obsessions and / or compulsions.

organic causality The concept that deviance is a function of organic cause such as brain injury, high fever, infection, virus.

organization That complex of relationships, both official and unofficial, which determine the manner in which any group will set about the achievement of its goals and objectives.

Pandora's box A mythological box containing all the ills and evils that could plague mankind; Pandora, a woman in Greek mythology, opened the box in spite of warnings not to, and released the ills and evils upon the world.

paranoia A type of disorder characterized by slowly developing, logical, well-systematized delusions of persecution and / or grandeur.

paresis General paresis; an organic psychosis caused by syphilitic infection of the brain.

patient-centered therapy A nondirective therapy developed by Carl Rogers which typically is neither as intensive nor as prolonged as psychoanalysis.

personality All aspects of a person which characterized his individuality and his relationship to others.

placebo Application of substances and procedures that have no demonstrable effect other than a person's belief that they do; the placebo effect is an improvement in the patient's condition or a change in the subject's behavior that occurs even though there has been no valid medication or therapy.

processes, unconscious Psychological processes or events of which a person is unaware; he does not verbalize the process.

prognosis A prediction regarding the future adjustment of a person in crisis.

program A set of activities pursued by an organization of persons based on a common set of goals, objectives, and tasks.

program development training project A system designed to facilitate program reorganization and to introduce training directly onto the treatment ward.

psycho surgery   Treatment of disturbed behavior by surgically cutting various nerve fibers in the central nervous system.

psychotherapy   Treatment of behavior disorders and mild adjustment problems through the application of personality theories and learning principles.

psychotropic medication   The various kinds of medications used in the treatment of disturbed thinking and behavior.

recidivism   The readmittance of a patient to an agency or institution.

remission   Marked improvement or recovery appearing in the course of a mental illness; may or may not be permanent.

restitutional therapy   A behavior modification technique where the patient is compelled to make good for his destructive behavior.

role   A set of behaviors or the perception of that set.

schematic   Pertaining to or in the form of a summary, diagram, or outline.

schizophrenia   A major psychotic disorder characterized by emotional blunting and distortion, disturbances in thought processes, and a withdrawal from reality. Army classification includes six subtypes: Latent, Simple, Hebephrenic, Catatonic, Paranoid, Unclassified.

self-actualization   According to Maslow, the highest need in man's hierarchy of needs.

seminal   Pertaining to or having the power of originality.

sheltered-care facility   A community residence for (usually) recently discharged mental patients which provides a somewhat structured and supervised living experience, often privately owned and operated for profit.

significance   Probability statement of the likelihood of obtaining a given difference of correlation between two sets of measurements by chance. Often stated by giving P values, for example, P<.001.

small group movement   The movement towards treating emotional problems in various types of groups rather than in individual psychotherapy.

snake pit   A popular term denoting conditions in the back wards of psychiatric hospitals.

social class   Grouping of people on a scale of prestige in a society according to their social status.

social group   Any formal or informal group of people who share some common interest or attachment and are characterized by face to face interaction.

social institution   A collection of objects, customary methods of behavior, and techniques of enforcing such behavior on individuals; for example, a union, mental hospital, army, political party, or school.

socialization   The process by which the family and culture teaches the child behavior they consider appropriate.

society   A group of individuals with a distinguishable culture.

somatic   Pertaining to the body; organic as distinct from psychological.

somatic treatment   Treatment consisting of physically or physiologically based techniques (drugs, surgery, electrical shock, etc.).

status   Position representing differences important in the exchange of goods and services and in the satisfaction of needs in a society.

subacute   The label for a dysfunctional person, either in a community or an institution.

synanon   A small group residential treatment approach to drug dependency.

team   An organization of persons whose existance owes itself to goals and objectives related to mental health service delivery.

technology   A specific plan or operation for effecting a change in an individual or a group, for example, behavior modification.

theory   In science, a principle or set of principles that explains a number of facts and predicts future events and outcomes of experiments.

therapy, supportive   Treatment of a personality problem by listening to a person's problems, suggesting courses of action, and reassuring him about what he has done or proposes to do.

tranquilizer   A psychotropic drug which relieves the symptoms of anxiety.

transference   The identification of someone in the immediate environment with some important person in that subject's past life.

trephining   An ancient treatment consisting of chipping or cutting a hole in the skull to release evil spirits.

turf   An area of responsibility within a system which is accompanied by authority and status.

validity   The extent to which a method of measurement does what it is supposed to do; validity is often expressed in terms of a coefficient of correlation representing the relationship between a set of measurement and some criterion.

References

Adler, A. 1924. *The practice and theory of individual psychology.* New York: Harcourt, Brace.

Agranoff, R., and Fisher, W. 1973. *Decision-making in mental health.* Paper presented at the Forum on the Politics of Mental Health, University of Illinois, Urbana, Ill.

Alexander, J.B., and Messal, J.L. 1972. The planning-programing-budgeting system in the mental health field. *Hospital and Community Psychiatry* 23:12.

Arnhoff, F.W.; Rubenstein, E.A.; Shriner, B.; and Jones, D.R. 1969. The mental health fields: an overview of manpower growth and development. In *Manpower for mental health,* ed. F.W. Arnhoff, E.A. Rubenstein, and J.C. Speisman. Chicago: Aldine.

Arnhoff, F.W.; Rubenstein, E.A.; and Speisman, J.C. 1969. *Manpower for mental health.* Chicago: Aldine.

Barton, R. 1959. *Institutional neurosis.* Bristol, England: Wright and Sons.

Belknap, I. 1956. *Human problems of a state mental hospital.* New York: McGraw-Hill.

Bleuler, E. 1911. *Dementia praecox oder gruppe der schizophrenien.* Leipzig und Wien: Franz Deuticke.

————. 1966. *Dementia praecox or the group of schizophrenias.* Trans. Joseph Zinkin. New York: International Universities Press.

Bond, E.O. 1954. Electroshock therapy: results of treatment in psychoses with a control series. *American Journal of Psychiatry* 110:881-87.

Braginsky, B.M., and Braginsky, D.D. 1973. Stimulus/response: mental hospitals as resorts. *Psychology Today* 6:10.

Brenner, M.H. 1967. Economic change and mental hospitalization: New York state, 1910-1960. *Social Psychiatry* 2:180-88.

352

Cannon, W.B. 1932. *The wisdom of the body*. New York: Norton.

Caplan, G. 1964. *Principles of preventive psychiatry*. New York: Basic Books.

Casriel, O. 1963. *So fair a house: the story of Synanon*. Englewood Cliffs, N.J.: Prentice-Hall.

Chu, F., and Trotter, S. 1972. *The mental health complex*. Part I: Community Mental Health Centers. Center for the Study of Responsive Law. Washington, D.C.

Coleman, J.C. 1972. *Abnormal psychology and modern life*. 4th ed. Glenview, Ill.: Scott, Foresman.

Cumming, J., and Cumming, E. 1962. *Ego and Milieu, the theory and practice of environmental therapy*. New York: Atherton Press.

Dancy, R.R. 1972. The broker: a new specialist for the community mental health center. *Hospital and Community Psychiatry*, vol 23.

Dunham, H.W., and Weinbert, S.K. 1960. *The culture of the state mental hospital*. Detroit: Wayne State Univ. Press.

Elinson, J.; Padilla, E.; and Perkins, M. 1967. *Public image of mental health services*. New York: Mental Health Materials Center, Inc.

Erikson, E.H. 1950. *Childhood and society*. New York: Norton.

Eysenck, H.J. 1966. *The effects of psychotherapy*. New York: International Science Press.

Fairweather, G.W. 1964. *Social psychology in treating mental illness: an experimental approach*. New York: Wiley.

Fenichel, O. 1945. *The psychoanalytic theory of neurosis*. New York: Norton.

Ferenczi, S. 1945. The brief analysis of a hypochondriac. In *Great cases in psychoanalysis*, ed. Harold Greenwald. New York: Balantine Books.

Fiedler, P.E. 1951. Factor analysis of psychoanalytic, non-directive, and Adlerian therapeutic relationships. *Journal of Consultative Psychology* 15:32-38.

Fisher, W. 1965. Social change as a therapeutic tool in a closed institution. *Psychotherapy* 2:3.

————. 1973. Incongruity between the university and the service agency. *Illinois psychologist*.

Fisher, W., and Laughlin, A. 1964. Observations on twenty patients who entered Elgin State Hospital in January, 1964. Unpublished manuscript, Elgin State Hospital, Elgin, Ill.

Fisher, W.; Mackie, R.; and Manelli, D. 1971. Proposal for reorganizing Elgin State Hospital: identifying needs and adapting to meet these needs. Unpublished manuscript, Elgin State Hospital, Elgin, Ill.

Fisher, W., and Mehr, J. 1965. A replication study, observations on twenty patients who entered Elgin State Hospital in January, 1965. Unpublished manuscript, Elgin State Hospital, Elgin, Ill.

Fisher, W.; Mehr, J.; and Truckenbrod, P. 1973a. Critical mass #1: treatment through institutional change. *JSAS Catalog of Selected Documents in Psychology*, vol. 3. p. 59.

————. 1973b. Critical mass #2: assumption, implications, and problem solving in treatment through institutional change. *JSAS Catalog of Selected Documents in Psychology*, vol. 3, p.89.

————. 1973c. *Power, greed, and stupidity in the mental health racket*. Philadelphia: Westminster Press.

Freud, A. 1945. *The ego and the mechanisms of defense*. New York: International Universities Press.

Freud, S. 1920. *A general introduction to psychoanalysis*. New York: Boni and Liveright.

————. 1930. *Three contributions to the theory of sex*. Nervous and Men-

353

tal Diseases Publishing Co.

—————. 1950. *Collected papers.* London: Hogarth Press.

Fulton J.J. 1951. *Frontal lobotomy and affective behavior: A neurophysiological analysis.* New York: Norton.

Garcia, L.B. 1960. The Clarinden plan: an ecological approach to hospital organization. *Mental Hospital.*

Glass, A.J. 1955. Principles of combat psychiatry. *Military Medicine* 16: 117.

Goffman, E. 1961. *Asylums.* Garden City, N.Y.: Doubleday.

Green, B. 1973. The little boy. *Psychotherapy: Theory, research and practice* 10:1.

Green, H. 1964. *I never promised you a rose garden.* New York: Holt, Rinehart, and Winston.

Hansell, N. 1968. Casualty management method: an aspect of mental health technology in transition. *Archives of General Psychiatry,* vol. 19.

—————. 1970. Introduction to the screening-linking-planning conference method (excerpts from discussions of triage problems). Unpublished manuscript, Northwestern Medical School, Chicago, Ill.

—————. 1970 Decision counseling method: expanding coping at crisis-in-transit. *Archives of General Psychiatry.*

Hobbs, N. 1964. Mental health's third revolution. *American Journal of Orthopsychiatry* 34:822-33.

Hollingshead, A.V., and Redlich, F.C. 1965. Social stratification and psychiatric disorders. In *Behavior disorders, perspectives, and trends,* ed. Ohmer Milton. New York: Lippincott.

Hull, C.L. 1940. *The mathematico-deductive theory of rote-learning: a study in scientific methodology.* New Haven: Yale Univ. Press.

—————. 1943. *Principles of behavior.* New York: Appleton-Century.

Illich, I. 1971. *Deschooling society.* New York: Harper & Row.

Jones, E. 1957. *The life and work of Sigmund Freud.* New York: Basic Books.

Jones, M.; McGee, R.; and Grant, J. 1952. *Social psychiatry.* London: Tavistock Publications.

Kasanin, J.S., ed. 1944. *Language and thought in schizophrenia.* Berkeley: Univ. of California Press.

Kennedy, J.F. 1963. Message from the President of the United States relative to mental illness and mental retardation. House of Representatives, Document 58.

Kirkbride, T.S. 1880. *On the construction, organization and arrangements of hospitals for the insane, Philadelphia.* New York: Arno Press.

Klein, Melanie. 1932. *Psychoanalysis of children.* New York: Norton.

Koestler, A. 1964. *The yogi and the commissar and other essays.* London: Jonathan Cape.

Kolb, L.C. 1968. *Noyes' modern clinical psychiatry.* Philadelphia: Saunders.

LeGuillant, L. 1946-47. Une experience de readaptation sociale institutee par les evenement de guerre. *Hyg. Men.* 36: 85-102.

Liefer, R. 1969. *In the name of mental health.* New York: Science House.

Lewin, K. 1935. *Dynamic theory of personality.* New York: McGraw-Hill.

Lindner, R. 1955. *The fifty-minute hour.* New York: Rinehart.

Low, A. 1950. *Mental health through will training.* Boston: Christopher Publishing House.

Martin, D.V. 1955. Institutionalisation. *Lancet.* 2:1, 188-90.

Maslow, A.H. 1940. *Motivation and personality.* 2nd ed. New York: Harper and Row.

Masserman, J.H. 1955. *The practice of dynamic psychiatry.* Philadelphia: Saunders.

McLuhan, M. 1964. *Understanding media*. New York: Signet.

McQuitty, L.L. 1938. An approach to the measurement of individual differences in personality. *Character and Personality* 7: 81-95.

Mehr, J., Truckenbrod, P., and Fisher, W. 1973. Core-competence training manual. *JSAS Catalog of Selected Documents in Psychology*, vol. 3, p. 90.

Mondale, W.F. 1972. Social accounting, evaluation, and the future of human services. *Evaluation*. 1:1

Moore, W.E. 1963. *Social change*. Englewood Cliffs, N.J.: Prentice-Hall.

Morgan, C.T. 1961. *Introduction to psychology*. 2nd ed. New York: McGraw-Hill.

Mowrer, O.H. 1953. *Psychotherapy: theory and research*. New York: Ronald Press.

—————. 1966. Integrity therapy: a self-help approach. *Psychotherapy* 3:3.

Murray, H.A. 1938. *Explorations in personality*. New York: Oxford Univ. Press.

National Institute of Mental Health. 1971. *Socioeconomic characteristics of admissions to inpatient services of state and county mental hospitals*. D.H.E.W. publications No. (H.S.M.) 72-9048, Superintendent of Documents, U.S. Government Printing Office. Washington, D.C.

Recovery, Inc. 1967. *Recovery, Incorporated*. The Association of Nervous and Former Mental Patients, Chicago.

Reik, Theodore. 1926. *Der schrecken*. Vienna: Psychoanalystischen Verlag.

—————. 1945. *The unknown murderer*. New York: Prentice-Hall.

—————. 1964. *Listening with the third ear*. New York: Pyramid Publications.

Rogers, C.R. 1942. *Client-centered therapy*. Boston: Houghton Mifflin.

—————. 1942. *Counseling and psychotherapy*. New York: Houghton Mifflin.

—————. 1961. *On becoming a person: a therapist's view of psychotherapy*. Boston: Houghton Mifflin.

Rogow, A.A. 1970. *The psychiatrists*. New York: Putnam.

Rosen, J.N. 1953. *Direct analysis*. New York: Grune.

Rowitz, L., and Levy, L. 1971. The state mental hospital in transition: an approach to the study of mental hospital decentralization. *Mental Hygiene* 55:1.

Russell, B. 1945. *A history of western philosophy*. New York: Simon and Schuster.

Sarbin, T.R. 1964. The concept of hallucination. *Journal of Personality* 35:3.

Scheff, T.J. 1966. *Being mentally ill: a sociological theory*. Chicago: Aldine.

Shakow, D. 1947. The nature of deterioration in schizophrenic conditions. New York: Nervous and Mental Disease Publications.

Skinner, B.F. 1938. *The behavior of organisms*. New York: Appleton-Century-Crofts.

—————. 1969. *Contingencies of reinforcement:* a theoretical analysis New York: Appleton-Century-Crofts.

—————. 1971. *Beyond freedom and dignity*. New York: Knopf.

Sobey, F. 1970. *The nonprofessional revolution in mental health*. New York: Columbia Univ. Press.

Specht, H. 1972. The deprofessionalization of social work. *Journal of the American Association of Social Workers* 17:2.

Spence, K.W. 1956. *Behavior theory and conditioning*. New Haven: Yale Univ. Press.

Stagner, R. 1948. *Psychology of personality*. 2nd ed. New York: McGraw-Hill.

355

REFERENCES

Stanton, A.H., and Schwartz, M.S. 1954. *The mental hospital.* New York: Boni Books.

Szasz, T.S. 1961. *The myth of mental illness.* New York: Hoeber-Harper.

————. 1970. *The manufacture of madness.* New York: Dell Publishing Co.

————. 1971. From the slaughterhouse to the mad house. *Psychotherapy* 8:1.

Truckenbrod, P. 1972. Training and human service systems in transition. Unpublished manuscript. Elgin State Hospital, Elgin, Ill.

Wexler, M. 1952. The structural problem in schizophrenia; the role of the internalized object. In *Psychotherapy of schizophrenia.* New York: International Universities Press.

White, R.W. 1948. *The abnormal personality.* New York: Ronald Press.

Wing, J.K. 1962. Institutionalism in mental hospitals. *British Journal of Social and Clinical Psychology* 1:38-51.

Yablonsky, L. 1965. *The tunnel back: Synanon.* New York: Macmillan.

Zilboorg, G., and Henry, G.W. 1941. *A history of medical psychology.* New York: Norton.

Index